In these

systems are compromised by the air we breathe and the food we eat, it is reassuring to know that there is at least one food which can actually reverse the effects of toxins—and that food is noni. According to Diana Fairechild, noni works on the body the way a good mechanic works on your car. It primes and balances your body to the point that the problem, no matter what the problem is, can no longer exist. With her compelling narrative style, Fairechild goes in search of the amazing noni; and where she goes is to the very heart of healing itself— to find not only the right medicine but also the right attitude for receiving the healing this medicine has to offer us.

Mysterious and ancient, noni has been used all over the world as a medicinal remedy for many diseases.

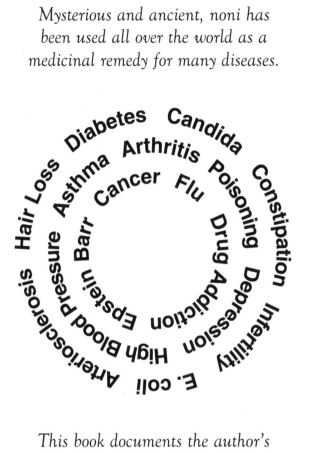

Diabetes Candida Arthritis Hair Loss Asthma Poisoning Arteriosclerosis Cancer Flu Constipation Barr Drug Addiction Depression High Blood Pressure Epstein Infertility E. coli

This book documents the author's use of noni to heal from the effects of pesticide poisoning and provides numerous other accounts of healing through the use of noni.

"It is early morning and I head down to the valley—looking for noni. *Thank you* I silently acknowledge each noni tree as I snap off the fruit. *Ba-bump* the fruit drums as I drop each piece into the bucket. *Ba-bump. Ba-bump. Thank you for being so fruitful even though no one is watering you. Thank you for healing me.* The morning light is increasing and the birds sing their exuberant welcome to this day. *Tweet-tweet woop-woop* I sing back mimicking their tunes. As I pick the noni fruit, the little bud faces smile and promise me that when I come back next week and next month there will again be plenty of fruit to harvest—plenty of noni for detoxification and healing."

—*Diana Fairechild*

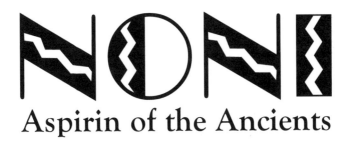

Aspirin of the Ancients

by

Diana Fairechild

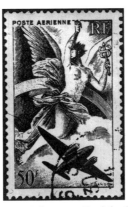

Flyana Rhyme Publishing

Copyright & Disclaimer

Flyana Rhyme Publishing
PO Box 248   Anahola Hawaii 96703—USA
    Tel/Fax: 808 828-1919
    Internet: http://www.flyana.com
    Email: diana@flyana.com

ISBN: 1-892997-81-9
Library of Congress Cataloging: 00-192885
1. Herbal Medicine 2. Detoxification 3. Hawaiiana

Kauai, Hawaii

JET SMARTER: The Air Traveler's Rx

The cabin of a commercial jet is one of the most sickening environments in the world. JET SMARTER offers an array of positive responses to the problem, changes in policies by the industry and also personal acts—defensive flying—that turn readers into smart flyers.

"The perfect gift for anyone who flies and a useful tool for business travelers."—*General Electric Corporate Newsletter*

"Take the advice of Diana Fairechild."—*Smart Money*

"Entertaining, meticulously researched."—*Business Traveler*

Office Yoga: At-Your-Desk Exercises

Prevent headaches, wrist problems, backaches and fuzzy thinking in 5 seconds to 3 minutes. Includes detailed illustrations and an extensive Symptom Chart.

"Required reading for anyone who works at a computer. Easy to do right at your desk and gives instant energy."

—*Carol McCullough-Dieter, Oracle8 for Dummies*

www.flyana.com
"Healthy Flying with Diana Fairechild"

Free information on the Web for airline passengers—on safe, efficient, healthy flying.

"Fairechild advises travelers of their rights."—*TIME Magazine*

"Engagingly personal series of columns."—*Los Angeles Times*

"One of twelve most creative Web sites."—*New York Times*

Table Of Contents

Photographs, Facts & Recipes

PHOTOGRAPHS

Facts & Recipes

This book is dedicated to the Hawaiian people with my deepest appreciation for keeping the ancient truths alive, which is an amazing feat considering their lack of a written language until 1820 and the plunder of their culture and lands. It is amazing that so much truth has survived for those of us lucky enough to reap what the ancient Hawaiian people have sown.

Noni Facts

Name: Noni, Indian Mulberry, and Morinda Citrifolia.

Market: Fruit and leaves.

Remedy: Modulates the immune system, laxative.

Native: South Pacific, India, Africa, Southeast Asia, Caribbean.

Habitat: At low elevations in the tropics and 100% sun brings larger fruit.

Planting: Transplant small trees, use cuttings and seeds.

Quirk: Ripe fruit smells like cheese.

Introduction

Feeling blue? Life got you down? Ancient natural medicine from Hawaii might be just what the doctor ordered.

Hawaii, long dependent on tourism and sugar, has found a new treasure buried in its own backyard.

Noni, prized by South Pacific islanders for hundreds of years for its natural healing properties, now looks set to join tea tree oil, St. John's Wort and aloe vera on the shelves of herbal wonder preparations.

Noni has been growing naturally in Hawaii's rich soil for generations and trees can be found in diverse climates from the wet streambeds on Kauai to the dry lava flows on the Big Island.

Juice from the fruit of the noni tree has been used to treat everything from high blood pressure to arthritis and infertility, and has even been linked to the control of cancerous tumors.

Now Hawaii's farmers are scrambling to catch up with rival noni producers in Tahiti and Samoa to supply a multimillion-dollar nutriceutical, i.e. nutrition as medicine, world market.

In ancient times, many Hawaiians had noni trees in their yards and drank the fruit juice as a cure for everything from influenza to senility.

In Hawaiian mythology, demigod Maui was restored to life after noni leaves were placed on his body. Volcano goddess Pele is also associated with noni, in that recent lava flows on the Big Island appear to have changed their course to spare old noni trees. One enormous tree in Kalapana, estimated at over 300 years old, has three ladders stationed around it for harvesting a year round bumper crop of noni fruit.

Today noni juice is prescribed by native healers for conditions ranging from high blood pressure, tuberculosis, arteriosclerosis, hair loss, and asthma to premenstrual syndrome, bee stings, jetlag, and detoxification.

Cancer research on the effects of noni at University of Hawaii in the departments of pharmacology and medicine has determined that noni seemed to suppress the tumor growth indirectly, by activation of the host immune systems.

It is only the shortage of available noni products that is presently restraining Hawaii's commerce in noni. Farmers are waiting for more noni trees to bear more fruit. Manufacturers have to turn away customers and they don't want to advertise because they don't have enough products to sell.

Some large plantings of Hawaiian noni will be maturing in the next couple of years. Farmers wonder among themselves if the worldwide demand for noni and other Hawaiian medicinals might eventually push agriculture to surpass tourism as the state's number one industry.

There is presently no testing for noni's potency. But healers on all islands agree that noni's potency is far greater when the plants are grown and the products prepared with traditional Hawaiian reverence and heartfelt prayers.

Perhaps tourism and agriculture will merge with planeloads of tourists coming to Hawaii for healing with fresh noni—along with our sunshine and the all-important aloha spirit.

Excerpted from a news article, "Remedy of the Gods," written by Diana Fairechild for Reuters News Service

Chapter 1

Healing with Noni

noninoninoninoninoninoninoninoninoninoni

The author learns
about the healing powers
of noni; but not before
she lost her health
and her livelihood.

noninoninoninoninoninoninoninoninoninoni

As an international flight attendant for Pan American World Airways and United Airlines, I logged ten million miles of air travel in twenty-one years. In an average month I crossed fifty time zones and missed ten nights of sleep. I was often on my feet for eighteen hours: pushing, pulling, reaching, serving, dodging and thinking ahead. Meanwhile, I had to look great, down to nail polish, spike heels and, in the early days, girdles.

The spike heels and girdles were uncomfortable. I was also uncomfortable being required to lie to passengers—squeezing my conscience into tight corporate image-shaping statements such as "of course your bags made it" and "the pesticide being sprayed in the cabin won't hurt you."

Towards the end of my career, I suffered terribly from the repeated pesticide sprayings on the aircraft, especially when I flew to New Zealand.

But I continued to fly—all the while my health deteriorating—until I was "medically grounded." I recall a number of personal warning lights that flashed before I had to stop flying.

On one of my last trips, after the cabin was disinsected [no misspelling*], I had temporary but nevertheless deep amnesia at the layover hotel.

Prior to each flight, the hotel operators call all crew rooms. "Pickup in one hour," the operators say. But oddly, that day, though I'd heard that specific phrase for two decades, what the operator was saying did not make any sense.

Pickup? Pickup? I faltered for a number of anguished moments. Then, glancing desperately around the hotel room, my uniform reminded me. *Oh! Pickup.* But the fear that I had temporarily lost a pathway to my memory haunted me from that moment on.

Memory lapses are not uncommon, of course. However it is neither common nor fitting for airline crew, who are responsible for the well-being and safety of the public.

I had to admit to myself that something was very wrong.

---

* "Disinsection" is the euphemism the airlines use for spraying pesticide in aircraft cabins and sometimes even right ON passengers. For more information, please see my book, *Jet Smarter: The Air Traveler's Rx*.

According to George Ewing, M.D., chief allergist at Straub Hospital & Clinic in Honolulu, the cause of my problem was my toxic workplace—the pesticides, secondhand tobacco smoke, and the recycled cabin air. Dr. Ewing explained to me that my workplace was poisoning me.

In the classic 1946 Alfred Hitchcock film, *Notorious*, the character played by Ingrid Bergman is being poisoned by her husband. The poisoning has a progressive effect: first, she simply doesn't feel well. Then, she becomes so sensitive to daylight she has to close all the window shades. Finally, she is bedridden. That's when Cary Grant arrives to save her.

That was Hollywood.

When I was medically grounded, I also became sensitive to light and had to retreat to my bed. Then, in order for me to get well—alas, with no Cary Grant to help me—I needed to revise my concept of "recovery," eventually agreeing to cultivate within myself peace of mind in spite of my health.

Prior to that decision, I imagined I would be able to get back the active life I had had before, as if in a fairy tale where all the good people live happily ever after with no net losses.

But new contexts and conclusions appeared in the tapestry of tales spun from the loom of my life; and the story of "The Princess and the Pea" became a personal parody.

. . . .*Once upon a time* there was a princess who got bruised from a pea under her mattress. All the kingdom praised her sensitivity saying it was her sensitivity that proved she was truly royal.

Actually, the princess could only tell the truth, and this proved that she was truly royal.

Years passed, and the kingdom became industrialized; and some people laughed when they heard the story of the princess. They whispered that she should toughen up.

One spring day the king decided to purchase the finest mattress money could buy and present it to the princess.

The mattress manufacturer knew he was about to make a killing. Everyone would want one of his mattresses once the princess said she'd finally had a great night's sleep.

In preparation for the First Night of True Repose, the court composer wrote a lullaby. Sweet cakes on doilies were placed on the princess's night stand, and a jasmine tree bloomed in full fragrance outside her window.

The bedroom door was shut. The whole country obeyed the king's decree for silence.

The next morning, a servant emerging from the royal chambers said: "The princess is ill. But it's not the pea this time—it's the chemicals they used to spray the mattress."

Mattresses are actually treated with toxic chemicals—allegedly to make them flea-free and therefore maintenance-free; and the princess was allergic to these toxins. Her eyes were puffy, she was achy, and she couldn't think clearly.

This was one princess who was not about to live happily ever after.

Pesticides Poison People, Too

. . . . My workplace—commercial jets—was routinely sprayed with pesticide while I was on duty. It lodged in my eyes and lungs.

In many airplanes today pesticide is still sprayed while the passengers cower in their seats with their seat belts fastened. Furthermore, all over the world, passengers get less oxygen to breathe than inmates get in U.S. federal prisons.

Researchers now blame chemical poisoning for many illnesses, though they go by a variety of names, including:

- Gulf War Syndrome
- Sick Building Syndrome
- Multiple Chemical Sensitivity (MCS)
- Environmental Illness
- TILT (Toxic Induced Loss of Tolerance)

In addition, neuro-degenerative diseases linked to toxins include: lupus, multiple sclerosis, Parkinson's, and Hodgkin's lymphoma. Even Alzheimers, while genetic, needs an environmental trigger. Autoimmune diseases such as rheumatoid arthritis and diabetes are also being traced to toxins. For starters, injuries caused by poisons weaken the immune system and leave people susceptible to other problems.

The workplace is often compromised with toxins. Though my workplace may have been different from yours, my story could be your story. Substitute a 747 for an office: new carpets and paint contain pesticides and air circulation systems are often inadequate.

45,000 people in the U.S. suffer every year from crippling injuries due to pesticide.[1] Champion ice skater Christine Locek was sunning herself in her yard one day when a lawn-care company sprayed pesticide at her neighbor's. The pesticide drifted towards her and her cat.

Within minutes Christine's cat was dead. The skater is now legally blind.[2]

"Lethal chemical drift" has been legislated in New Jersey, Florida, Colorado, Connecticut, Louisiana, Maryland, Michigan and Pennsylvania. In those states, lawn-care companies are required to notify people—only people who ask, that is—twenty-four hours before pesticiding within a half-mile of their home.[3]

When I was medically grounded in 1987, I did not know what to do. What I now know I hope will light the way for others. Because I was living in Hawaii when I became ill, and some Hawaiians were kind enough to share with me what they knew, I have learned a little about traditional Hawaiian healing.

I am comfortable taking noni because it has a long history of successfully treating humans, it is completely natural, and when I drink noni juice I can actually *feel* it working.

Noni is the most widely used medicinal herb in Polynesia. The Hawaiian word for "herb" —la'au—refers to the entire plant: fruit, flowers, bark, roots, and leaves. It is an honor for me to share information about the *la'au,* noni, that is making me well.

Diana's Recipe to Prevent & Eliminate Toxic Poisoning

1. **Minimize exposures to toxins.** Avoid, whenever possible, toxins such as dry-cleaned clothes, new carpet, perfumes, and chlorinated pools. If you exclude what you can, your system may not get overloaded, the way mine did.

2. **Recharge the body.** Strengthen your organs daily with physical exercise, a healthy diet, and heartfelt gratitude.

3. **Detoxify.** Remove poisons by drinking substantial quantities of clean water and eating herbs such as noni.

Chapter 2
Basic Immunity Building

noninoninoninoninoninoninoninoninoninoni

Suggestions for how
to be aware of
and strengthen
the immune system.

noninoninoninoninoninoninoninoninoninoni

Would you believe me if I told you I can see my immune system?

If you want to see your immune system, look for it when you do things that strengthen it such as spending time outdoors in Nature, and when you do things that weaken it such not drinking enough water and not doing what you really feel like doing.

Seeing the immune system requires only a simple shift of focus similar to the way we can shift our eyes from a foreground object to a background object.

My immune system first became visible to me when I fell ill. It looked like a suit of armor that was cracking up. I was in such in a highly sensitized state, that even news on the radio brought me to tears.

One day, however, what I heard on the radio did not bring me to tears—instead it turned on a light in my brain. The broadcast I was listening to concerned a chemical commonly found in many household products including spray paint. It is called 1-1-1—and the announcer said it was ruining the ozone layer.

At that moment, it seemed to me that just about everything I was allergic to was also ruining the ozone layer; and my mind extrapolated that because of my sensitivity I had become a bellwether for the ozone layer.

This realization removed my pall of self-pity for being a victim of chronic illness. From that moment, as I became enthusiastic about my potential for playing a role in improving the ozone layer, my health recovery accelerated.

My enthusiasm touched on all things that benefit from a healthy ozone layer—pristine air, the oceans, all species. Love for life grew in me.

I believe that enthusiasm for anything in your life will strengthen your immune system.

I saw a dog yesterday. His head was out the window of a car that barreled down the road at top speed. The dog's open jaw seemed to be set in a smile. The look on the dog's face could only be described as enthusiastic!

I was on my way to the health food store and the produce manager had that same look on his face when he was extolling a specific variety of avocado.

"Nothing's as good as the Sharwils," he said enthusiastically.

It is this pure joy which fortifies the immune system.

What is the joy that will heal you? Have you ever heard the birds sing at dawn? They sing their hearts out. *Here comes the dawn.*

Joy is a universal cure-all. Dare to chirp your own song—be true to your own inner longings. You may find them at first in small ways—the satisfaction of repairing the torn hem of a favorite garment or of adding a new gizmo to your mountain bike.

As we all unleash our own joy, we help the world at large by our example. Every feeling of joy repairs the "ozone layer" of our minds.

Some day, people will realize that the ozone layer of our planet is affected as much by the pollution of our minds as by the pollution in our bodies.

Great joy shimmers brighter than the sun reflecting on the sea—brighter than any glitter paint.

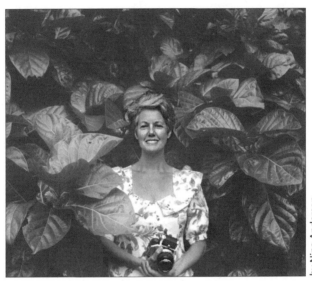

by Nina Anderson

Diana with Old Nikon & Old Noni

I live in a remote area of Hawaii where there are thousands of noni trees. I am a lifelong vegetarian and yoga practitioner. Born in New York, I graduated from Boston University after spending a year at the Sorbonne in Paris. My next twenty-one years just flew by as an international flight attendant. It was during those years that I settled in Hawaii.

Chapter 3
Going With The Flow

noninoninoninoninoninoninoninoninoninoni

Surf the self
and experience
the bliss of
awareness.

noninoninoninoninoninoninoninoninoninoni

Going With The Flow

Most of my flying years were spent with Pan Am, based in California. I often flew around the world in eight days. My layovers were in London, Beirut, Delhi, Bangkok, Hong Kong, Tokyo and Honolulu.

Hawaii was always a place where I could unwind, and I found the people especially kind. My oldest friend from those days, Peter, still lives near Honolulu.

Peter and I share a love for the ocean. "I've never had a swim I didn't like," she says, coaxing me if I get wishy-washy about jumping in when the sun is not bright or the water just-right.

One windy day I was stung by a man-o-war, which is a jellyfish that can drift in close to shore. The sting on my arm started screaming with alarm, as though I had stuck it in a flame and could not pull it out. Peter took me to her friend Peggy's house, because it was nearby and Peggy had aloe growing in her garden.

"Interesting that you should show up today," Peggy said when she saw me. "Our neighbor's guest cottage just became available. You said you love this place. So if you ever thought of moving here, this would be the time."

The cottage came with a 180-degree view of Lanikai Bay, often frequented by TV commercial producers because of its picturesque offshore islands. I could rent it if I wanted, the landlady said. I called Pan Am. "As a matter of fact," a cheery voice told me, "Honolulu is short-staffed, so you can transfer in right away."

I felt stunned—first the man-o-war sting and now this astonishing thing—I couldn't tell if I felt good, excited, flattered, frightened, or what. "I don't know why," I told Peter, "but I'm having a hard time saying 'Yes.'"

"If you move to Hawaii, you'll be going with the flow," Peter commented.

I had never thought of life as having a flow, a current like the ocean. Until that moment, I'd done pretty much what my parents, teachers, lovers, and employers had wanted me to do. Fear of offending had motivated me. Now, for the first time I decided to let the flow carry me to Hawaii.

Years scrolled by. I worked for Pan Am in the Pacific until Pan Am left the islands and United Airlines hired me. After two years with United, I was medically grounded.

A couple of months later, my landlady's son wanted the Lanikai cottage, and my doctor advised me to move to an even more unpolluted place. I found a cabin at the 3000-foot elevation on Maui and lived there for seven years until a new neighbor with a huge stereo moved in.

I moved to Hana. The house I rented there was toxic and I couldn't find another quiet perch on Maui. I found one on Kauai.

Meanwhile, I absorbed myself in activities whenever I felt the flow. I got busy helping airline passengers demand fair and conscientious treatment by the airlines. Helping others helped me to feel better.

So, I am still in Hawaii, the surfing capital of the world. Though I've never taken a board to the sea, it feels as though I've learned to surf by proximity. The first principle is this: paddle in the same direction as the wave you want to catch. To move to Hawaii, I got my job transfer, packed up my favorite things, took a leap of faith, and paddled hard—going with the flow.

Great surfers, I learned, don't even need to paddle. When a great wave comes, they stand up at the exact right moment and "drop in." It's the moment when the wave is ready and strong.

Surfers tell me that riding waves makes them very aware, in effect, super-conscious. The ride becomes a magnified mirror of their inner personality. Balance is the only way through. Neither ego nor denial works. If they deny their own power, they cannot keep up and they lose the wave. If they overstate it, they get ahead of themselves and lose it, too.

One choice leads to the next. It is not possible to control the situation. In the power, surrounded by the wave, they enjoy the ride for as long as it lasts. There are no mistakes. Yes, there are risks. It's about trust. And it is also a lot of fun. In fact, it is bliss.

Once I heard about this bliss, I had a strong desire to learn to drop into my own wave—the wave called my life. And then a big wave came for me to practice on—although it didn't seem so big at the time. It came in the form of a flock of chickens, escaped from their pen, seeking asylum at my mountain sanctuary on Maui. Their raucous clucking interrupted my peace. . . .

How annoying. *Cock-a-doodle-do.* I can't think. *Cock-a-doodle-do.* I can't write. I'll call the Humane Society. If I catch the roosters, the Humanes will take them away.

NONI by Diana Fairechild

They bring a cage. It's really for dogs. They set the trap, then leave. *Squawk squawk.* I catch a hen and two chicks. The chicks shimmy through the wires and scramble away. The hen cries, screams nonstop while I wait for the Humanes. I ignore the cries and try to write.

Thump. Thump. Two peacocks land on my porch. Their claws are twice as big as my fingers! Their attention is singular. They stare into my eyes. I hear the hen's cries—and more. Roosters and chickens are now surrounding my cabin; they all chorus the hen's cries.

"Okay!" I tell the peacocks. I walk outside and release the hen. She runs free, still crying. I go back inside and lie down.

The *cock-a-doodle-dos* are not annoying now. It actually sounds as if the roosters are saying something in English. What is it? I know, it sounds like "Re-mem-ber God." "Re-mem-ber God" "Re-mem-ber God." I remember. And I am in bliss.

"Thank you," I silently tell the roosters. *Their instant silence confirms that I have indeed dropped in.*

The following poem by William Blake, the English mystic and poet, elucidates so elegantly what I mean by "dropping in."

"To see the world in a grain of sand,
And heaven in a wild flower;
To hold infinity in the palm of your hand,
And eternity in an hour."

Dropping in is the balance place, neither so far outside the energy of nature that we miss it altogether, nor so far inside the chaos of its force that we are damaged in the tumult. One of the most important components of dropping in is the willingness to wait for great waves. I've learned that waiting for a great wave requires patience—that it is a time to refine listening skills, to heighten awareness of distant waves from afar before they shape up into view.

There have been many blissful times with smooth rides and the relationship with the waves understood and managed—times of proficiency and synchronicity when the practice begins to pay off. There have also been many times when I've misjudged the waves, and crashed on sharp coral reefs. Sometimes the reefs scraped me pretty badly. I have also had to swim among sharks (in my ten-year court battle with United Airlines). In spite of these challenges, I keep picking myself up and getting back on my board. I think of my board as my intention. It's not always easy, but it's the way the flow leads me. It's the Hawaiian way.

Hawaiians invented surfing. There's something special in the spirit of a people who choose to transmute the awesome, sometimes destructive energy of waves, into fun. Imagine, too, the attitude that guided the Hawaiians to experiment with herbs like noni.

How many times I must have walked past noni trees unaware of the answers they offered to my blind imbalance. How many places I looked before I saw what was right before me. How appropriate that the noni tree be common, unnoticed, and generous with its deep shade—and that its fruit, the ambrosia of health, be UNsweet and rich with the earthy aroma of natural process.

When I'd finally struggled enough, noni was there for me, giving in abundance. By the seashore—under a noni tree—I was led to the bliss of my healing processes. I am grateful to the Hawaiian people for placing this fruit in my hand.

My healing work with noni is another graceful step along a wondrous path called Life. Perhaps I have finally found the balance point, the right relationship to life on Earth. If so, then my private symbol for this relationship is noni.

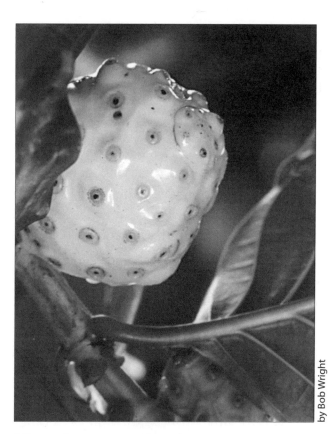

by Bob Wright

Noni Ready for Picking

Noni is ready for picking when the color of the fruit is yellowish-white.

NONI by Diana Fairechild

Chapter 4

On the Path to Noni

noninoninoninoninoninoninoninoninoninoni

The author is led
through ancient
sacred grounds
to her first encounter
with the noni.

noninoninoninoninoninoninoninoninoninoni

On the Path to Noni

My noni journey started at an airport—the tiny airport in Hana, Maui—but it was not for a flight. Kahalewai and I were hiking the Kings' Trail. He wanted to show me an important Hawaiian artifact.

We skirted the runway until we reached the coast. The trail then disappeared into a jumble of giant black lava boulders and I was having trouble walking. This was no garden path. Sometimes there was no foothold, only ridges of sharp lava to perch on. The facets on the stones faced every which way.

Kahalewai, though older than I and weighing over 220 pounds, appeared graceful as a ballerina as he leapt from boulder to boulder.

Wondering about my stamina, I began to say, "I am afraid . . . . if I fall . . . ."

Kahalewai stepped back and took my hand. As I teetered to one side, he leapt to that side to keep me from falling. He gracefully escorted me across the uneven terrain.

After an hour or so Kahalewai stopped. I thought it was a rest stop, so I sat. I noticed as I relaxed that the stones under me were all about the same size, actually small like pebbles, and the area was flattened at the top, definitely a design of some sort. "What's this?" I asked, pointing.

"Grave. No point at grave."

I saw then that Kahalewai was standing by another grave. I jumped up thinking I shouldn't be sitting on a grave. As I got up, I felt an odd surge of energy, as though a fresh spring inside me had just been loosed from a dam. I recalled feeling just this way, otherworldly, in Machu Pichu in Peru, but I had credited that to the high altitude. At this moment, however, I was at sea level. The feeling was the same, though. Very peaceful. Very empty of thoughts and desires.

Kahalewai smiled. "Ancestors," he said, gesturing with his eyes. I could almost see his ancestors—tall with regal bearing.

We lingered until the dimming light reminded us it was time to move along. We did not backtrack to the airport, but continued along the coast in the same direction towards a park where we had left Kahalewai's car. (A friend had dropped us at the airport.)

The trail hugged the bays and inlets of the coastline winding to the whim of the land and the sea. Around another bend we saw the famous black sand beach, Waianapanapa, sprinkled with tourists in colorful bathing attire—an opulent tapestry of swimsuits and towels with the black sand as a background making all the colors worn by the tourists appear especially vibrant.

The trail then descended in a switchback to the beach. Kahalewai bounded across the little beach in a couple of strides.

As I joined him on the other side, he drew me into the shade of a large tree with big shiny green leaves shaped like spades in a deck of cards. White, yellow and green fruits hung artfully like ornaments on a Christmas tree. The aroma—both fruity and cheesy at the same time—reminded me of a first-class cheese and fruit cart on the airplane.

Kahalewai plucked a white fruit about the size of a large apple and placed it in my palm. I had never seen this fruit before. The fruit's skin had a translucence like human flesh and it seemed to have big goose bumps all over it.

"This is noni," Kahalewai said. "Noni heal me. Two friends die after we work with pesticide in the fields. I sick, very sick. Auntie give me noni. I give you noni. It heal you."

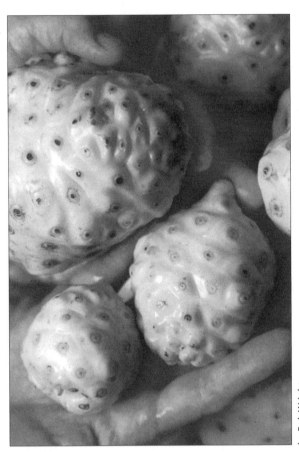

by Bob Wright

NONI FRUIT WITH HANDS

This noni was just harvested as a crop.

Chapter 5
A Pesticide Antidote

noninoninoninoninoninoninoninoninoninoni

Kahalewai offers his
family recipe
for preparing
and using noni
as an antidote for
pesticide poisoning.

noninoninoninoninoninoninoninoninoninoni

Kahalewai's Noni Recipe for Pesticide Poisoning

1. Pick the noni fruit when it is white, but still hard. Let it ripen in the shade. "The mature fruit is the healer; we call it *o'o* in Hawaiian," says Kakalewai.

2. Massage the noni through a strainer to remove the seeds.

3. Put the pulp in a glass jar in the sun for a day. Then refrigerate.

4. Take a tablespoon in the mornings. "Everything is according to how you feel. If you feel good, keep taking it. If you feel nothing, but okay, keep taking it," says Kahalewai.

NONI by Diana Fairechild

A Pesticide Antidote

Kahalewai is 100% Hawaiian. His family is *ali'i*, Hawaiian royalty deposed and dispossessed. They lost all their land in his grandparents' time because they did not pay taxes on it. His grandparents were unable to read English, and apparently did not even know they had to pay taxes on their land. There never had been land taxes when Hawaii was populated only by Hawaiians.

Once the white settlers came from the mainland, they introduced taxes; and they also introduced the alphabet. During this period, in the earliest written history of Hawaii, noni trees are prominently mentioned, specifically during The Great Mahele, the land apportionment by King Kamehameha in 1845. At that time, the Hawaiian people were permitted to petition the king for small parcels of land if they could show they had been improving the land. Many Hawaiians claimed they had improved their land by cultivating noni.

The Great Mahele marks the beginning of land ownership in Hawaii—even by the king. Prior to that, all the land in Hawaii belonged to the gods.

In 1845, according to Frances Frazier, eleven thousand claims for land were filed. Ms. Frazier has translated all of them from Hawaiian to English for the Hawaii State Archives, and she told me that a large percent of the claims cited noni as one of the ways people said they had improved their land.

In fact, cultivation of noni was referred to more often than any other way, she said, by Hawaiians at that time who were claiming that they had improved their land.

I asked Ms. Frazier to translate the meaning of the word "noni."

"Noni," she said mysteriously, "is an ancient name. It is time out of mind. No one that I know of knows what it means and I certainly don't know how it can be translated."

Chapter 6
The Common Cold

noninoninoninoninoninoninoninoninoninoni

Two Hawaiians
choose to take
noni's healing properties
into their own hands.
One shares his recipe for
nipping a cold
in the bud.

noninoninoninoninoninoninoninoninoninoni

DAVID'S NONI RECIPE
FOR COLDS

1. Pick the softest noni fruit on the tree. "Fruit so ripe you hold your hand underneath and it drops into your hand like it was waiting to serve you," says David.

2. Mix the fruit in a blender.

3. Strain the seeds and skin.

4. "Drink all the pulp you can right away."

AUNTIE ROSANNA'S NONI
RECIPE FOR COLDS

1. Chew a handful of noni flowers.

2. Spit out the flowers.

The Common Cold

David was brought up on Kauai. His ancestors are Hawaiian, Chinese, Irish and German. When David feels as if he's coming down with a cold, he says: "My nose feels stuffy. Gonna get a cold. Gotta drink noni."

Linda works as a tour bus driver on the Big Island. She collects tourists at the airport about 8 a.m., drives them around all day, then gets them on a 5:30 p.m. flight back to Honolulu.

One day a sneezing tourist rode in her bus. He said he also had a sore throat. At 10:30 a.m., at the City of Refuge, Linda pointed out a noni tree and told him that the local people eat this fruit when they have colds.

This tourist took one bite of a ripe noni and spit it out. "It smells!" he screamed.

About an hour later, at Volcano House, Linda noticed that this tourist was no longer sneezing. At 5:00 back at the airport, she asked him, "How's your cold?"

He had "totally forgotten about it," he said.

"Hawaiians they smart, huh?" Linda teased.

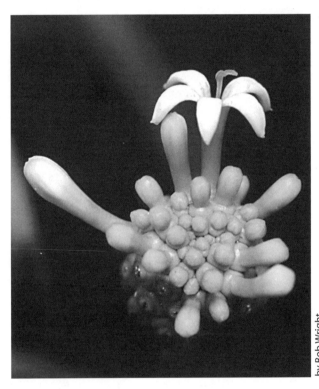

by Bob Wright

Noni Flower

The noni flower is botanically "perfect" containing both pollen-bearing (male) and ovary-bearing (female) parts.

Chapter 7
Pain Relief

A few topical uses
of noni including
its application to joint
and muscle injuries,
rashes and skin sores.

noninoninoninoninoninoninoninoninoni

Nina's Noni Recipe for Sore Joints

1. Pick the softest fruit on the tree.

2. Squish the fruit with a potato masher.

3. Warm your skin with a hot towel so that it will accept the noni's healing.

4. Smooth on the noni.

5. There's a comforting feeling as you cover your skin with the noni. When the comforting feeling goes or the ache returns, rinse your skin with fresh water, then smooth on the noni again.

Pain Relief

Nina tapes compresses of noni pulp to her swollen joints. She trains horses, and has been thrown a number of times.

Nina has lived on Kauai for thirty years, originally coming here from California.

Her friend, Alice, was confined to a wheelchair, leaning to one side because of the pain in her spine. Nina smeared noni pulp on Alice's back every day. Alice drank noni juice every day, too. After five weeks, Alice's pain began to leave and she could sit up straight.

I've also had a remarkable experience using noni fruit topically. Four years ago I had a deep cut on my leg when a nail from a packing crate gouged my skin. The cut was about two and a half inches long, and I probably should have had stitches, but I didn't.

For awhile, every time I drank noni juice, the wound began to hurt, as if it were saying to me, *I want noni too.* So I dabbed the wound with fresh noni fruit and the ache stopped immediately to my amazement.

The wound has now completely healed and the scar has smoothed out and faded.

NONI by Diana Fairechild

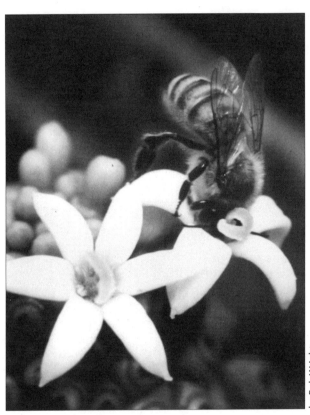

by Bob Wright

BEE INTO NONI FLOWER

The delicate scent of noni flowers invites bees into the pollination process.

Chapter 8

Aphrodisiac

noninoninoninoninoninoninoninoninoninoni

A European
living in Hawaii
drinks noni wine
and says it enhances
his sex life.

noninoninoninoninoninoninoninoninoninoni

GREG'S RECIPE FOR
NONI WINE

1. Pick the noni fruit when ripe.

2. Put the fruit in a covered plastic bucket in the sun for three or four days.

3. With a small hose, siphon the fermented juice into another bucket, leaving the sediment at the bottom of the bucket.

4. Put the fermented juice into a covered glass jar out in the sun for several more days.

5. Open the jar occasionally so the impurities can run over.

NONI by Diana Fairechild

Aphrodisiac

A popular legend has it that noni was brought to Hawaii in canoes from Tahiti. There is another legend, though, that noni was here long before the Tahitians came. This ancient account describes a continent in the Pacific called Lemuria which predated Atlantis and which also sank.

The Hawaiian Islands are what is left of Lemuria, the tips of an ancient mountain range, according to this older legend. And it is said that for the Lemurians noni was an aphrodisiac.

An aphrodisiac is something which "arouses or increases sexual desire."[12] and a neighbor of mine, Greg, drinks noni wine for just this reason. He's originally from Europe and his preparation for noni is patterned after wine making. Greg is in his seventies. When asked about noni, Greg beats his chest and says, "With noni I will live to one hundred!"

The term aphrodisiac may also encompass love in a broader sense. There are people I've spoken with who experience a lightness of being when they eat or drink noni fruit—a lightness that they say opens them to love and kinship with all humanity and with all life.

NONI by Diana Fairechild

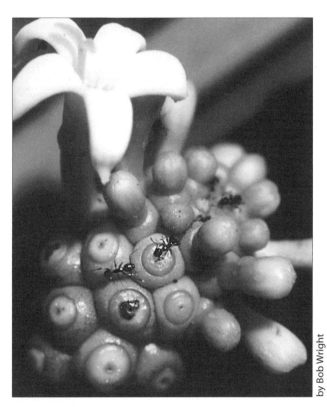

by Bob Wright

Noni with Ants

Ants crawl around on the "eyes" scavenging nectar after the flowers have dropped.

Chapter 9
Intestinal Worms

noninoninoninoninoninoninoninoninoninoni

Hawaiians
keep pet care
costs down.

noninoninoninoninoninoninoninoninoninoni

Noni Remedy for Worms in Animals

1. Mix the noni into the animal's food; approximately one piece of fruit or its dried equivalent per meal per animal. One piece of fruit equals 15 to 20 capsules depending on the size of the fruit and the dosage of the noni caps.

2. If you are using dried noni from a capsule, add water to it first before mixing it into the pet food.

3. Anecdotally, noni is very effective for worms; however, it is advised to first start with a small amount, no larger than one serving, and observe the results.

"This is how we avoid expensive bills at the vet. The vet is *sooo* expensive," a local woman at the grocery store told me. She was about eighteen years old.

I had asked her if she knew about noni. She smiled and said that her father feeds noni to their seven hunting dogs.

"Once a month, or sometimes whenever you know the dogs are getting sick because they're not as lively and the color of their *doo-doo* is dark black, and sometimes you can even see the worms come out of it. Also, if the dog is not gaining weight, something is wrong, then we mash the ripe noni, about half and half, right into their dog food."

"What kind of dog food?" I asked her.

"Dry dog food with water," she said, adding, "It is very well known that noni cures worms."

Like other nutritional protocols, which have been developed for animals and then are later implemented for humans, noni appears to be an efficacious remedy for worms and parasites, in humans as well as pets.

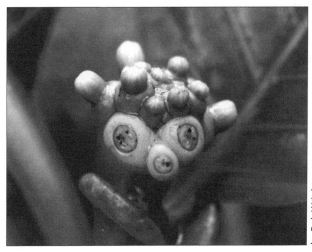

by Bob Wright

Noni Bud Face

As tiny flowers bud, the noni begins to resemble an extra-terrestrial. The antennas (buds) reach for the sun. After noni flowers wither and drop, marks are left on the skin of the fruit. In Hawaii, we call these markings the noni "eyes."

Chapter 10
Long-Term Illness

noninoninoninoninoninoninoninoninoninoni

Two grandmothers
drink noni juice
to recover from
chronic illness.

noninoninoninoninoninoninoninoninoninoni

Nani's Noni Recipe
for Diabetes

1. Pick white, hard noni. "Not too ripe," Nani says, "because the very ripe fruit has bugs."

2. Wash the fruit and let them ripen in the kitchen.

3. Mix the noni in a blender to apple-sauce consistency. Strain the seeds; use a fine-mesh strainer because the seeds are small. Refrigerate.

6. "I drink two jiggers of noni pulp before bed at night and again two jiggers first thing in the morning," says Nani.

NONI by Diana Fairechild

Nani Saffery, a 78-year-old *kupuna* (respected elder) takes noni instead of insulin for diabetes.

"I drink two jiggers of noni pulp before bed at night and again two jiggers first thing in the morning. I remember my grandmother gave us the ripe fruit from the noni tree. As we grew older these things were forgotten. After I was told I had diabetes, I remembered noni and I started drinking it. A year later I was tested again for diabetes, and I no longer had it. It's been twenty years now."

Similarly, Nancy, a 63-year-old, 300-pound Hawaiian was diagnosed with high blood pressure twenty-five years ago. Nancy has been drinking noni for high blood pressure for two decades.

Nancy drinks noni juice every morning for two weeks and then abstains from the noni for about a month. She feels the noni cleans her out and reduces all her symptoms of high blood pressure.

Then the abstaining time is important, too, as it gives her body time to fully absorb the medicinal benefits of the noni.

NONI by Diana Fairechild

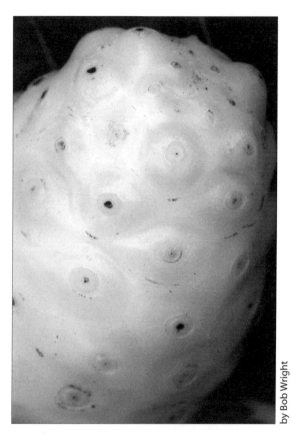

by Bob Wright

Ripe Noni

With white translucent skin, this very ripe noni smells like ripe, French cheese.

NONI by Diana Fairechild

Chapter 11

Autism

It might be good
to "back off"
even when you're
making progress
with noni.

Vici is autistic. She is six years old. Her parents started giving her noni about five months ago. After two days of noni, Vici's attention span doubled and her parents were delighted.

"I think noni juice is great stuff," her father told me. He's an air traffic controller and he's also taking the noni. "At first," he continued, "I thought the noni gave me a false energy, like speed, because I had so much more energy than before.

"But now, after five months, I realize it's not like speed at all because I'm feeling so much better across the board."

Vici was given noni every day, too, and she even started talking, something which 50% of autistic children never do.

Autism is a developmental disability that typically becomes known to parents during the first three years of their child's life. Autism effects the brain and the child's ability to concentrate, typically with difficulties in verbal and nonverbal communication. Since Vici was improving, especially her attention span, her parents kept Vici on the noni juice, one ounce a day.

But then, suddenly, after about three months on noni, Vici started getting daily nosebleeds. Vici hadn't been doing anything else new, so her parents stopped the noni.

A couple days later, the nosebleeds stopped.

Vici's Dad told me, "Maybe the noni is a blood thinner like aspirin. Noni has helped Vici a lot and I would like to stay with it if I can because I believe it helps Vici to make progress. And whatever she learns, she retains."

Vici is not so scattered when she's taking noni, she's able to generalize, her energy level is high, and she keeps improving, her Dad explained.

After two months off noni, Vici is now going back on. I suggested smaller doses this time, and also less frequency, following the advice of the Hawaiian elders I had interviewed. (See the next chapter.)

Vici's new dosage is now one teaspoon of noni first thing in the morning three times a week.

I also suggested that her parents keep a log with dates, dosage and their observations, so others may benefit as well.

Chapter 12
Noni Healing Protocols

noninoninoninoninoninoninoninoninoninoni

Several approaches
to developing a personal
healing protocol
with noni.

noninoninoninoninoninoninoninoninoninoni

Every Hawaiian I've ever met knows about noni. Young people do not much favor the fruit because of its cheesey smell; but elders greatly value noni and each appears to have his or her own prescriptive recipe for the best way to prepare and take the noni. Here are some of the comments I've heard:

"Just a tablespoon of noni juice with meals." "Noni only works when drunk first thing in the morning." "People with heart conditions should not drink the noni that grows near the ocean because of its high salt content." "You gonna get holes in your stomach by drinking too much noni."

In Hawaii, many "local" people also refer to traditional protocols for taking noni. For example, Linda, the Big Island tour bus driver, described the protocol of her 75-year-old father-in-law, a native of Kauai of Portuguese descent whose parents came here as laborers for the sugar plantation. Since his prostate cancer surgery eight years ago, noni is part of his morning routine. He dilutes the juice with water and drinks it once a day for three days, then stops for two days.

An elder, local woman I met at the beach while she was on her way back from picking seaweed from the offshore reef near where I live, told me that she drinks noni only on the odd-numbered days of the month, such as the 1st, 3rd, etc.

I have found, in connecting with people in the Hawaiian community—and there's no total agreement about this—that the tradition of backing off is typical. It appears to me that all the traditional formulas have rhythms that include backing off in some manner. But it's not talked about in this way. For example, some local people take the noni only for two days, then they don't take it on the next two days.

The traditional rhythms have been a starting place for me—maybe because I'm the kind of person who finds it hard to stick to recipes in cookbooks. When I follow a traditional formula and observe what is happening in my body and my emotions, then I feel I know intuitively how I want to experiment on my own.

Lyons Naone, a *kahuna*, or expert, on Maui, told me he personally uses noni to help with jetlag, and he recommends noni to those who need a cleansing, such as after holidays when there's been a lot of overeating and drinking. Noni helps them to "clean out and get back on track."

Naone tells his patients who want to do more than just a seasonal or after-travel cleanse to drink noni for five days, then abstain for the next five days. The five on, five off rhythm can be maintained until the problem is cleared up, "whatever the problem may be."

Peter Waldo, a microbiologist, brought his microscope over one day and we looked at noni juice. "A budding yeast and an abundance of bacteria" is what we saw. "Yeast, of course, is seen on the skin of Brie cheese in a totally safe fermentation," Peter said. Anyway, I felt good a few minutes later when Peter gulped down all of the noni juice I brought him. It was the first he ever drank and he said he liked the taste.

That was not the case with me. At first, I didn't like the taste of noni. The cheerleading of Kahalewai goaded me on. As I began to feel better, though, the taste also grew on me. My affection for noni reminds me of the way friendships grow. After sharing enjoyable experiences with someone, their appearance changes for me—people become more attractive as I become fond of them.

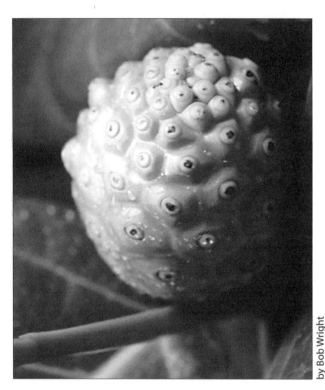

by Bob Wright

GREEN, OR UNRIPE, NONI FRUIT

Fruit grow in the direction of the sun with the older eyes smoothing out towards the bottom.

Chapter 13
Green, or Unripe, Noni Fruit

noninoninoninoninoninoninoninoninoninoni

Numerous traditional
applications for
unripe noni; and
an experiment with
unripe noni has an
unusual result.

noninoninoninoninoninoninoninoninoninoni

USES OF GREEN, OR UNRIPE, NONI FRUIT

"Use the green fruit...for sprains, injuries, pain."

—R.M. Heinicke[9]

"For deep cuts squeeze juice from the half-ripe fruit onto the area."

—B. Krauss[10]

"Unripe fruit is mashed and mixed with salt, then applied to skin for bone breaks" and "mashed and applied to the head for concussions."

—I.A. Abbott[11]

Green, or Unripe, Noni Fruit

Luckily for us, the ancients experimented with noni and learned what works. If not for them, we might remain asleep to all the possibilities.

Anthea, a woman I know with chronic health problems, did not want to try noni because of the smell. So one day we decided to make juice from the odorless green fruit. We washed a dozen noni, then put it through a juicer; it got real foamy and Anthea said it looked like "a root beer float."

The taste was sweet, more like apple juice or possibly persimmon juice, than the pungent ripe noni juice I am used to.

I drank two big glassfuls. There is a tendency to overdo sometimes, especially when you've been ill and you think you've found a cure. Suddenly, I felt very tired, as if I'd hit a wall. I went home, crawled into bed, and slept for three days! Anthea had only one glass and she said she was fine.

I found no mention of this kind of experience in my research, though I uncovered many medicinal references to the green, or unripe, noni fruit. Some are included on the facing page.

There are many accounts of the drawing out property of noni fruit used topically including this remarkable report from 1972 recounting how a U.S. military officer stationed in Hawaii successfully used noni fruit:

"A naval officer's only remaining hurdle to a promotion was a physical examination which he had been dreading because of the painful inflammation of a sprained elbow. Green noni fruits were mashed with salt into a poultice for the elbow. Next morning the elbow was healed and the officer passed his exam and received his promotion."[8]

Another anecdotal use of green, or unripe, noni fruit is its drawing out property for bee stings and mosquito bites.

Additionally, some old noni hands in Hawaii, swish the first sip of noni around in the mouth and then spit it out, claiming this helps to remove toxins in the mouth, such as those caused by dental work including mercury fillings.

Chapter 14
Native Healing

noninoninoninoninoninoninoninoninoni

Native healing
practices involving
noni and other herbs
are now coming
to the forefront in
alternative medicine.

noninoninoninoninoninoninoninoninoni

O NONI EYES

O noni eyes.
You have 118 eyes on all your sides.
I have two—maybe three eyes.
I want to truly See.

You remind me of the all-seeing
Creator
Who blesses us with the Truth
And educates us to heal.
To You who put noni on the earth,
Thank you.

Help me to unwind the skein
Of complex abuses,
My own energy misuses,
That left me Unfree.
Please heal me.

NONI by Diana Fairechild

The missionaries in Polynesia outlawed spiritual healing in 1879—under penalty of a stiff fine. This obviously did not stop natural healing because in 1915 another law was enacted, and this time the penalty for accessing the supernatural was imprisonment!

Still today, however, natural and supernatural healing flourish in the Hawaiian Islands, and wellness and prayer are intertwined.

"It isn't a matter of just swallowing noni juice and it's all okay," said *kahuna* Naone. "Prayer is part of the healing. There is no set prayer. The prayer is according to what the illness is, who is being treated, and what the situation is."

What prayer of long ago led me to the noni tree? The noni fruit's multiple eyes remind me to open my own eyes—outer and inner—to the possibilities of answers and blessings coming from any direction. I pray for willingness to accept healing from whatever direction it comes.

On the opposite page is my noni prayer.

Chapter 15
Noni & Cancer

noninoninoninoninoninoninoninoninoninoni

Noni's role in
fighting cancer.
Researchers throughout
the world confirm what
native people have
always known.

noninoninoninoninoninoninoninoninoninoni

Noni & Cancer

A University of Hawaii botanist who did not wish to be quoted told me she has had a lot of calls from people who say noni cures things like cancer tumors, kidney problems, and hair loss. One person called her, she said, claiming noni cures high blood pressure. Another called and said noni cures low blood pressure. To the botanist, that proved people just don't know what they are talking about. However, this information about both high and low blood pressure fits with the theory that noni may be an immune system modulator and overall body balancer and, as such, it can heal the body no matter what the health problems are.

In many countries, noni is considered the "tree of life" because its fruit, flowers, leaves, roots, bark and seeds all offer people free medicine for good health and longevity.

In support of this, there is a huge body of research on noni that goes back many generations in many cultures. "Traditional remedies have been selected over generations for efficacy by trial and error," explains a research paper from the Indonesian *Journal of Ethnopharmacology*.[13]

Here are a few noni remedies from the above mentioned Indonesian journal.

Abdominal pain: drink boiled noni fruit.
Diarrhea: drink mashed noni seeds.
Fever: place noni leaves on the body.
Mental illness: eat the skin of noni root.

A 1951 Filipino research paper presents thirty-two uses of noni from around the world. Here are some of the highlights:[14]

Anti-arthritic: sap of leaves (Philippines).
Carthartic: roots (India).
Diarrhea: char the leaves (India).
Cleansing: fruit is a shampoo and also cleans iron and steel (China).
Colic: apply heated leaves to the chest (Malaysia).
Fever: drink tea from the bark (Congo).
Food: cook young leaves (Java), eat the fruit with salt (China).
Spongy gums: rub gums with charred unripe berries mixed with salt (India).
Tonic: leaves, bark and stems are pounded, cooked and strained and then drunk (no specific region).
Ulcers: apply the leaves (Philippines).

A researcher in Tonga,[15] references noni specifically for women's health issues:

> **Breast hardness after childbirth**: drink an infusion of noni leaves.
>
> **Infertility**: the couple should drink tea from noni bark.
>
> **Painful urine**: the woman should drink an infusion of noni leaves.

Another researcher in Tonga[16] touts noni as the "most widely used medicinal plant of ancient Polynesia" and cites these traditional uses:

> **Mouth infection**: eat ripe noni fruit.
>
> **Stomach ache**: infusion of leaves or bark.
>
> **Sty**: noni flower sap when first broken off.
>
> **Evil spirits**: drip an infusion of noni leaves into the eyes, nose and throat.

Thirty-two years ago, the Hawaii Medical Association meeting opened with the following prophetic phrase: "Ancient Hawaiian knowledge is enjoying a sudden rebirth of interest."[17] At the conference, noni was referred to as a favorite remedy for two totally different conditions:

> **Hypertension.**
>
> **Tiredness in old age.**

"Antibacterial Properties of Some Plants Found in Hawaii,"[18] a paper published fifty-one years ago by researchers at the University of Hawaii Department of Bacteriology, documents noni's efficacy against these three bacterial agents of disease:

> **Staph:** ripe fruit.
> ***E. coli***: ripe fruit.
> **Typhoid bacillus**: unripe fruit.

A book by University of Hawaii researcher Beatrice Krauss,[19] published in 1993 by the University of Hawaii Press, lists medicinal properties of noni's flowers and fruit for:

> **Boils.**
> **Kidney and bladder disorders.**
> **Constipation.**

A paper on the medicinal plants used by Hawaiians, published in the 1985 *Journal of Ethnopharmacology*,[20] describes how noni has been traditionally used in Polynesia for:

> **Asthma.**
> **Fractures.**
> **Skin infections.**
> **Sprains.**

In the Cook Islands, noni root is put on top of the head to treat stonefish stings. In Tahiti, noni fruit is applied directly to stonefish stings.[22]

R.M. Heinicke, a pineapple researcher in Hawaii, published a paper in 1985 called "The Pharmacologically Active Ingredient of Noni." Heinicke credited noni's healing properties to an enzyme he termed "xeronine." In order for xeronine to work, the noni fruit must be taken on an empty stomach, Heinicke said, otherwise the "pepsin and acid in a stomach digesting food will destroy the enzyme."[23]

In 1979, two Department of Chemistry scientists, one from the University of Hawaii and the other from University of Guam, found caprylic acids in noni fruit.[21] Caprylic acids are known for controlling yeast fungus.

In 1993, Japanese researchers discovered that an extract of noni root inhibited Epstein-Barr virus and suppressed a cancer gene.[24]

This supports anecdotal evidence in the islands about noni curing cancer.

I met with a 79-year-old man on Kauai, Masashi, who told me he's been drinking noni sun tea since his stomach was removed fifteen years ago because of cancer.

"I take one jigger of noni juice in the a.m. and one jigger in the p.m.," Masashi said, adding, "The strength of the noni is not in the juice alone. You gotta get the sunlight, at least two days in the sun."

Masashi has dozens of gallon jars of noni in his yard. He gives the juice away to anyone who shows up at his door, free of charge.

He also told me he is hoping someone with AIDS comes by to try his noni. He's hoping noni will help AIDS patients as much as it's helped him and other patients with cancer.

At the American Association for Cancer Research 1992 meeting a paper was presented on noni. It found that ripe noni juice significantly prolonged the lives of mice that had cancer.

The paper said: "It [noni] seemed to suppress the tumor growth indirectly via activation of host immune system."[25]

Activation of the immune system may be what is apparently curing cancer. Research is continuing.

Chapter 16
Be Your Own Physician

noninoninoninoninoninoninoninoninoninoni

The Truth
is behind
the eyes.

noninoninoninoninoninoninoninoninoninoni

DIANA'S RECIPE FOR
NONI SUN TEA

1. Pick the noni when it is hard.

2. Wash the fruit and let it ripen in the fresh air. The fruit is ripe when it is soft to the touch, translucent to the eye and cheesey to the nose.

3. Fill glass jars with the ripe fruit, cover tightly and place in the sun.

4. Leave the jars in the sun for a couple of days or up to a year.

5. Strain the juice to remove the skin, pulp, and seeds. Refrigerate.

6. Drink one ounce on an empty stomach.

NONI by Diana Fairechild

Be Your Own Physician

I enjoy drinking noni juice and in Hawaii, I prepare the juice myself. Many people in Hawaii prepare noni fruit juice simply by putting the ripened noni in glass jars and then letting the sun do the work, making in essence, a sun tea. One *kahuna* says you can leave the noni in the sun for up to a year[4] and I've found that the longer it's in the sun, the better I like the taste.

Making noni sun tea, the noni "eyes" separate from the skin and float off in the liquid. One morning, alone in my house, as I sipped my noni drink, I noticed that there was a noni eye in my glass. While I took small sips to avoid getting the eye in my mouth, I thought I heard a voice, possibly an incoming call on my answering machine, but it wasn't the phone.

Then I heard the voice again, now more distinct. "I'm glad you like me. I like you," it said.

"Who are you?" I asked, looking around.

"I'm the noni eye in your glass."

"If you are speaking, please wink," I said.

The eye didn't wink. But the little voice spoke up again in rhyme: "I don't wink. Some say I stink. I'm a great drink. I can think."

NONI by Diana Fairechild

"What are you thinking?" I replied.

"I'm thinking, I like you more than you like yourself." I didn't say anything. We sat together quietly like a couple of old friends who don't feel the need to talk.

"I always make you feel better, right?" the eye scolded. "You sometimes do things that don't make you feel good—like eating that quart of ice cream last night."

"What's in ice cream?"

"There's refined sugar, of course. That's come up in tests as something that really hurts the immune system. The immune system recognizes sugar as a friend, but it is an impostor. When the energy from the sugar wears off, your body can lurch. Eating large quantities of sugar may be okay, occasionally, for hardy folks. Energy blips are minor for them. But not for you."

We sat in silence again until the eye spoke. "You know, ice cream is full of antibiotics, the ones that are given to the cows, of course. People are dying in hospitals these days because they have become antibiotic-resistant; so when they get sick, there are no drugs that work—all from eating factory-farmed animal products filled with drugs and growth hormones to fatten them up."

"That's horrible!"

"Come on," said the eye. "You know all this, but you're blinded because in your childhood ice cream always made you feel good. We heard your prayers. We want to turn your health around. *We are doing all we can.*"

"What are you doing?"

"We work on your body the way that product in the auto parts store works on your car, prolonging the life of the engine, upgrading its fuel economy, filling in any light scratches in the cylinder walls and puting a protective film over all lubricating parts. Once you like yourself as much as we like you, you will really see improvements in your health."

I enjoy drinking noni juice—even when I'm having a busy day and don't have time to listen to the noni.

Indeed, I find that it is nothing short of astounding that there can, and sometimes is, a subtle communication coming from the spirit of the noni plant. I certainly believe drinking noni juice has helped me to know myself better.

With self knowledge you can be your own physician. It is free, and it is freeing.

NONI by Diana Fairechild

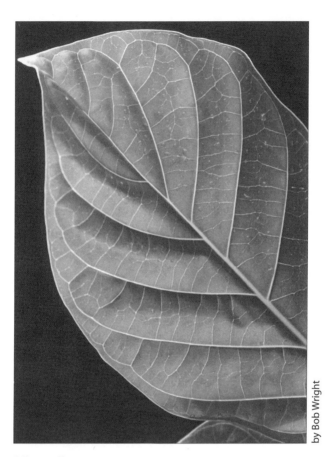

by Bob Wright

NONI LEAF

In Java, noni leaves are served as a vegetable.

Chapter 17

Noni Leaves for Rashes, Arthritis, Swelling & Immunity

noninoninoninoninoninoninoninoninoninoni

Noni leaves are
used externally and
internally.

noninoninoninoninoninoninoninoninoninoni

Naone's Recipe for Noni Leaf Tea

1. Pick yellow leaves from the noni trees. Most of the leaves are green and there are just a couple of the yellow leaves here and there. If possible, pick the leaves only at sunrise.

2. Wash the leaves.

3. Bring the leaves to a boil in a large pot of water, then simmer for twenty minutes.

4. The more leaves you use and also the longer you simmer the leaves, the stronger the tea will become.

5. Strain and drink.

Noni Leaves for Rashes, Arthritis, Swelling & Immunity

In one account of Polynesian mythology, the god Maui was restored to life after noni leaves were placed on his body. This myth shows how noni leaves were believed to be restorative—and possibly even divine—by the ancient Polynesians.

In Polynesian healing, you consider the two distinct sides of noni leaves, the top side (which basks in the sun) and the bottom side (which faces the earth).

It is the top side of noni leaves that can heal us, according to *kahuna* Naone.

"The top side is called *alo*, which means 'facing the sun.' The sun gives the leaf the power to heal," Naone told me.

"Noni leaves can also be drunk as a tea to boost the immune system," Naone added. "Here the leaves should be picked at sunrise because this is internal medicine. Always pick the yellowed leaves right off the tree; the entire leaf should be yellow for preparing tea for the immune system."

Leaves intended for external uses—such as for rash, arthritis or swelling—should be picked at sunset. "External medicine is picked and prepared at sunset," explained the *kahuna*.

Noni leaves range in sizes comparable to human hands—from small children's hands, to medium-sized women's hands and big men's hands. Some of the older trees have leaves larger than basketball players' hands.

The University of Hawaii botanist who did not believe that noni fruit could regulate blood pressure does believe the leaves are as good as any antibiotic for infected cuts.

A research paper called "Medicinal Plants of the Philippines" also has great praise for noni leaves: "It is not uncommon throughout Malaysia to heat and apply the leaves to the chest or to the abdomen for coughs, enlarged spleen, nausea, colic and fever."[14]

Noni leaves have helped me to get rid of a painful rash that erupted at the base of my spine after my landlord pesticided around the base of my house the year I lived in Hana, Maui. Over the next four months, the rash spread up and across my back; it lasted until several weeks after I'd moved from that toxic environment.

Six months later, after a low back injury, the rash erupted again. It felt like constant stinging needles. I put a noni leaf on my back to see if it would help and the stinging subsided quickly.

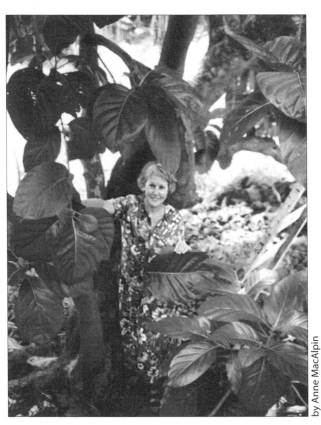

by Anne MacAlpin

Diana with Kalapana Noni

This 300-year-old noni tree has big leaves and as much shade as a banyan. See ladder on right.

I left the leaf in place and the rash did not spread that day. There were no new eruptions the next morning so I kept another leaf on my back all the next day and night again. The following day the rash was gone.

To release the healing power in the noni leaves some people heat them over a flame. I like to bathe with a few leaves in very hot water. This softens leaves and also makes the bath water medicinal. When I get out of the tub, I towel dry the leaves then place them on my body overnight. It's a very comforting feeling when the skin is inflamed.

As for how to make the noni leaf tea, here's what I recommend when people ask me how many leaves to use and how long to boil them. I would start with a partial leaf steeped for only fifteen minutes and see if you like the taste of the tea. Then wait a few days to see if the tea has any medicinal effect on you. Do this for several days and observe what you experience. If you like what's happening, you may want to increase your dose. Of course, continue to observe yourself and be sure to consult your doctor.

Chapter 18

Detoxification

noninoninoninoninoninoninoninoninoninoni

How cleansing
the immune system
with noni fruit
compares to detoxifying
in a sauna.

"Detoxification" means to remove toxins, or poisons, from the body. Toxins can accumulate in the body from a lifetime of commonplace activities such as eating pesticide-treated food, sleeping on a chemically-treated mattress, and wearing dry-cleaned clothes. Chemicals in baby mattresses are now tracked to a majority of cases of Sudden Infant Death Syndrome[26] and the dry-cleaning solvent perchloroethylene is a known bladder carcinogen.[27]

We can also accumulate toxins suddenly in large crippling doses, as I did from the routine pesticiding which takes place on commercial jetliners. Similar health problems as mine afflict the men and women who served in the Gulf War. Their uniforms were apparently saturated with pesticide in a skewed belief that this would prevent the troops from having to deal with lice!

Detoxifying with noni can and should be done very gradually so that even sensitive types like me can tolerate it. Nevertheless, I would like to make it clear that detoxifying is definitely not glamourous.

Sometimes old symptoms stir up; in this sense, it could appear that there are side effects. For example, the headaches I used to have when I was working on jets sometimes reactivate during periods of detoxification. As the body eliminates damaging chemicals stored in the fat cells and soft tissues, old symptoms can reactivate and old food cravings may kick in, as well.

After much experience with this kind of thing, I now regard these so-called "side effects" as indications that my body has started to detoxify— a good thing. At the onset of side effects, I try to remember that what is really going on is detoxification and secondly, the best course is to back off from the noni for awhile.* When I follow this strategy, periods of setback are shorter and less intense.

My personal regimen of "human detoxification," as it is called in environmental medicine, also includes saunas accompanied by high doses of niacin, a B-vitamin supplement.

Niacin creates an internal heat that apparently helps the toxins move out of fat cells and into the bloodstream where the additional

---

* See "Noni Healing Protocols" on page 81

heat of the sauna induces perspiration to permanently excrete the toxins.

Noni also creates an internal heat and initiates a detoxification, although it is much subtler than the sauna method.

Sauna detox is a well-known therapy for chemical poisoning, and once I heard about it, I wanted to try it. I got my chance a couple of years ago while I was living on Maui.

A woman named Brenda thought I'd be the perfect person to endorse her Sauna Detox Program. Brenda waived the $1,300 fee in exchange for my potential endorsement and she invited me to use her newly built sauna on the other side of the island from where I was living.

I declined, however, not feeling up to a daily two-hour drive. Long trips in traffic pollution did not make sense to me while detoxifying.

A few weeks later Brenda called to say she had met Jason who lived near me and he had a sauna at home. Brenda offered to oversee both our programs, which she expected would take about two weeks. Brenda always liked to pair people up, she told me, so that her clients would watch out for each other in case of heat stroke or dehydration.

It was in this context that Brenda wanted me to call Jason my "twin."

The purpose of sauna detox is to eliminate through sweat the toxins that prevent the body from functioning optimally.

Brenda told me about a woman who had been dyeing her hair black for decades. During the detox, black dye oozed out of the pores of her arms.

Brenda also talked about a man who had been exposed to asbestos. During the sauna detox his back broke out in welts. These were analyzed in a lab and found to contain minute traces of asbestos fiber. In both cases, Brenda said, the detox was "turned on" by the sauna's heat along with high doses of niacin.

The woman with the black-dyed hair, the asbestos worker, and thousands of other people had stayed in the sauna until their symptoms vanished. They were cured, Brenda said with confidence.

My doctor had actually heard of this program and he gave the okay. So I committed to baking naked four hours per day at 140-degrees with a man I had only just met for as long as it would take to eliminate of all my symptoms.

It was Brenda's and my hope that this would cure me of my ills.

Jason wanted to detox from decades of recreational drugs. He has a cedar sauna with a TV monitor for a window, so I rented us a couple of videos each day on my way to his house.

For three weeks we sweated together and we took niacin starting the first day at 50 mg. and ending three weeks later at 3200 mg.

In retrospect, I feel it is not productive to detox in a sauna with others because it is inevitable that we will breathe in and absorb through the skin some of the poisons that others are releasing. It can also be emotionally challenging.

During our time together, Jason had a herpes outbreak and he also had an LSD flashback. People who take drugs are known to experience "flashbacks" and to exhibit a "drug personality" during detoxification,[28] and dealing with Jason's personality was a problem, especially when I was in my own healing crisis.

In the heat of our extended moments in the sauna, I had to continually fend off Jason's advances. I never did call him my twin, and I had no interest in sharing a womb experience with him.

The symptoms that showed up for me during the sauna detox were almost unbearable—to the degree that every other part of my life had to shut down.

Brenda explained that my symptoms indicated high amounts of poisons being eliminated.

Here is a partial list of what I experienced during the three-week sauna detox: back pain, gall bladder pain, swollen junky eyes, dizziness, headache, random and severe itching, slurred speech, and intense light sensitivity. It was the staph infection, however, that motivated me to stop the program. The open sore on my arm got larger and deeper each day.

I've had staph a number of times, it being common in the tropics, and I felt it was impossible to heal from the staph infection while my skin stayed wet with daily four-hour saunas. I did not want to take antibiotics because of allergic reactions I have experienced in the past, so I decided to stop the sauna detox program on the twenty-third day.

A month or so later the staph on my arm healed using herbs.

Nevertheless, I am glad I got to do the sauna program; I believe I derived benefited from it. During my healing crisis I experienced myself as more authentic and after a six months' recovery, I was stronger than before the program.

Still, I do not believe in crash-and-burn detoxification.

Within the detox circles I have traveled in, sauna is much touted as the way to go for swift and complete detoxification. My experience proved otherwise.

If possible, detoxification should be gradual, natural, and personally guided.

What I like better about noni as a detox path is that noni is slower and more controlled, more gentle, more private, and it doesn't take as much time.

Healing is very personal. Everyone has an individual experience, an individual threshold at the inner space of knowing oneself.

Healing is about following your heart, following your gut feelings and being responsible to yourself. These are as much the ingredients of the remedy as the medicine itself.

For me, the answer lies in healthy, conscious living and an ongoing relationship with a divinely-given assistant. Noni.

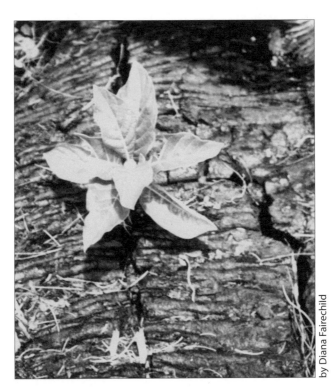

by Diana Fairechild

NEW NONI IN A LAVA CRACK

Noni self-propagates on hardened lava starting about seven years after the molten lava erupts.

Chapter 17

Table of Referenced Uses for Noni

noninoninoninoninoninoninoninoninoninoni

Noni has been used
in traditional and modern
medicine for a wide array
of illnesses and injuries.

noninoninoninoninoninoninoninoninoninoni

HINTS FOR USING THE TABLE

1. *References*
   The far right column of the Table gives the names of referenced sources. The small numbers following these references refer to the Endnotes, which are consecutively numbered beginning on page 173.

2. *Multiple Noni Parts*
   For some diseases or conditions, more than one part of the noni plant has been recommended.

3. *Not Available* (n/a)
   Some of the references do not specify how to use the noni.

Table of Referenced Uses for Noni

Starting on the next page, the "Table of Referenced Uses for Noni" includes a list of health conditions in the left-hand column with corresponding noni uses to the right.

The Table is compiled from the work of many researchers–both ancient and contemporary, mainstream and obscure, funded and unfunded.

The oldest reference is from a 1922 publication from Territory of Hawaii entitled: "Hawaiian Herbs of Medicinal Value Found Among the Mountains and Elsewhere in the Hawaiian Islands, and Known to the Hawaiians to Possess Curative and Palliative Properties Most Effective in Removing Physical Ailments."

Spanning every decade since that publication in the 1920's, the "Table of Referenced Uses for Noni" cites dozens of books and papers, as well as some anecdotal sources where this seemed appropriate and helpful.

I hope this "Table of Referenced Uses for Noni" will be of some value to you in your healing and I will continue to update it in the future.

Condition	Noni Part(s)	Method(s)	Reference
Arteriosclerosis	green fruit	juice & drink	Heinicke [9]
Arthritis	green fruit	juice & drink	Heinicke [9]
	leaf sap	apply/pained area	Quisembing [14]
Asthma	n/a	n/a	Abbott [20]
Backache	fruit	boil w/water, drink	Elliott [13]
Beriberi	fruit	juice & drink	Quisembing [14]
Bladder	flowers/fruit	n/a	Krauss [6]
Boils	ripe fruit	mash & apply	Krauss [6]
	unripe fruit	cut in half, apply	Handy [29]
	leaves	heat & apply	Handy [29]
Bones, Broken	young fruit	mash w/salt, apply	Handy [29]

Condition	Noni Part(s)	Method(s)	Reference
Burns	green fruit	n/a	Heinicke [9]
Cancer	ripe fruit	juice & drink	Hirazumi [25]
	root extract	drink	Hiramatsu [24]
Cancer, Breast	leaves	poultice	Singh [15]
Cathartic	root	n/a	Quisembing [14]
Colds	n/a	n/a	Abbott [20]
	ripe fruit pulp	drink	anecdotal
Colic	leaves	heat, apply/chest	Quisembing [14]
Concussion	unripe fruit	mash, apply/head	Quisembing [14]
Constipation	n/a	n/a	Krauss [6]
Cough	leaves	heat, apply/chest	Quisembing [14]

CONDITION	NONI PART(s)	METHOD(s)	REFERENCE
Cough (continued)	fruit	juice & drink	Quisembing [14]
	bark	n/a	Handy [29]
Cuts	seeds	mash & apply	Handy [29]
	young fruit	pound w/salt, apply	Kaaiakamanu [30]
Depression	green fruit	juice & drink	Heinicke [9]
	skin of root	pound & drink	Elliott [13]
Diabetes	ripe fruit	mix w/water, drink	McBride [31]
	ripe fruit	boil juice, drink	Handy [29]
	ripe fruit	mash to pulp, drink	anecdotal
Diarrhea	seeds	mash w/water, drink	Elliott [13]
Diarrhea, Infant	leaves	char w/mustard	Quisembing [14]

Condition	Noni Part(s)	Method(s)	Reference
Digestive Problems	green fruit	juice & drink	Heinicke [9]
Drug Addiction	blossoms	eat/5 days	Handy [29]
Drug Addiction	green fruit	juice & drink	Heinicke [9]
Dysentery	leaves	char	Quisembing [14]
Epstein-Barr	root	extract & drink	Hiramatsu [24]
Evil Spirits	leaf infusion	rub on body	Whistler [22]
	leaf infusion	drip into eyes/nose	Whistler [22]
Fever	bark	n/a	Quisembing [14]
	leaves	heat, apply w/oil	Elliott [13]
Gout Pain	leaves	apply to pain	Quisembing [14]
Gum Disease	berries	char w/salt, apply	Quisembing [14]

Condition	Noni Part(s)	Method(s)	Reference
Heart Disease	ripe fruit	ferment & drink	Handy [29]
High Blood Pressure	green fruit	juice & drink	Heinicke [9]
Hypertension	ripe fruit	ferment & drink	Handy [29]
Hypoglycemia	ripe fruit	mash, eat w/meals	Tabrah [5]
Infertility	unripe fruit	eat	Anecdotal
Inflammation	bark infusion	couple drinks daily	Singh [15]
Indigestion	leaves	poultice	anecdotal
Insect Bite	n/a	n/a	Abbott [20]
Kidney	ripe fruit	apply	Anecdotal
	flowers & fruit	eat	Krauss [6]
	ripe fruit	poultice	Quisembing [14]

CONDITION	NONI PART(s)	METHOD(s)	REFERENCE
Laxative	ripe fruit	mash w/sugar, drink	Quisembing [14]
Liver	fruit	juice & drink	Quisembing [14]
Menses Cramps	unripe fruit	juice & drink	Heinicke [9]
Mouth Infection	fruit	juice, apply/mouth	Whistler [16]
Nausea	leaves	heat, apply/stomach	Quisembing [14]
Old Age	ripe fruit	mash, eat w/meals	Tabrah [5]
Pain	green fruit	juice & drink	Heinicke [9]
Senility	unripe fruit	juice & drink	Neal [7]
Skin Infection	unripe fruit	juice & drink	Krauss [6]
	leaves	crush or char/poultice	Abbott [11]
Skin Rash	ripe fruit	juice/mist skin	anecdotal

CONDITION	NONI PART(s)	METHOD(s)	REFERENCE
Shigella	unripe fruit	n/a	Bushnell [18]
Sore Throat	fruit	syrup/gargle	Quisembing [14]
Spleen, Swollen	leaves	heat, apply/spleen	Quisembing [14]
	fruit	juice & drink	Quisembing [14]
Sprains	unripe fruit	add salt, apply/sprain	Stewart [8]
Stomach Ache	bark or leaves	make infusion, drink	Whistler [22]
Stonefish Sting	root	grate, apply/crown	Whistler [22]
	fruit	apply to sting	Whistler [2]
Sty	leaf petiole	apply	Whistler [22]
Tonic, Old Age	leaves & bark	pound/cook/strain	Quisembing [14]
Tonic, Childbirth	fruit	boil w/water, drink	Elliott [13]

Condition	Noni Part(s)	Method(s)	Reference
Tuberculosis	fruit	n/a	Quisembing [14]
Typhoid	ripe fruit	n/a	Bushnell [18]
Ulcers, Gastric	ripe fruit	juice, drink w/water	Stewart [8]
Yeast Fungus	dried fruit	n/a	Levand [21]

Noni's ability to effectively address all of these above conditions may be, in part, due to Noni's known antibacterial and antibiotic properties:

Condition	Noni Part(s)	Method(s)	Reference
Antibacterial	ripe fruit	juice & drink	Levand [21]
Antibiotic	ripe fruit	juice & drink	Bushnell [18]

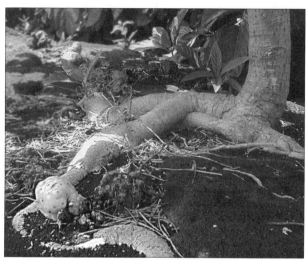

by Diana Fairechild

NONI ROOTS

On the Big Island, noni roots travel above the ground seeking cracks in the hardened lava before they penetrate downwards towards a water source.

Chapter 20
Where Noni Grows

noninoninoninoninoninoninoninoninoninoni

The where, when
and how of noni.

noninoninoninoninoninoninoninoninoninoni

NONI by Diana Fairechild

Noni trees thrive throughout the world in in a broad range of tropical ecosystems. In the Hawaiian Islands, noni roots dig right into the rigid lava on the Big Island, Hawaii's newest island, and also flourish along the many streambeds of Kauai, Hawaii's wettest island.

Noni trees also grow along the ocean coastlines on all Hawaiian islands in the gritty soil just inland from sand; and here their big leaves get tattered from the salty tradewinds.

Near my home on Kauai, thousands of noni trees grow in a quiet valley that opens to the ocean. This valley gets about fifty-five inches of annual rainfall. Twelve months a year this valley has a bumper crop of noni.

Mature noni fruit can be both smaller than a golf ball and larger than a baseball. As a matter of fact, both large and small fruits grow on the same trees at the same time. The trees in full sun bear more fruit—and larger fruit—than those under the forest canopy.

Even young trees just 18 inches high (about 18 months old) bear fruit.

NONI by Diana Fairechild

When classifying trees like noni, botanists compare primarily the tree's flowers, not the medicinal properties of the plant. Noni is classified in the botanical family Rubiaceae, which also includes coffee trees. When I learned that noni and coffee are in the same botanical family, however, I began to wonder if the immune system support offered by noni might be likened to the stimulation of coffee.

I find that the after-effect of drinking noni juice is definitely less intense than drinking coffee—noni feels more like a steady hum as compared to the buzz of coffee. And I tremendously enjoy the feeling of warmth as the noni makes its way down to my stomach. The warmth then radiates throughout the rest of my body, even to my hands and feet. I used to have cold hands and feet, but never, since I've been drinking noni juice.

Other names for the noni tree are Indian mulberry, Morinda citrifolia, nonu, nono, bumbo, lada, munja, and canary wood. By any name, noni is respected and revered as an immune system modulator—bringing the body into balance by adjusting and adapting the protective field around and within us and by varying the body's vibrational pitch and intensity, as necessary.

NONI by Diana Fairechild

Chapter 21
How Noni Looks

noninoninoninoninoninoninoninoninoninoni

In successive stages
of maturation, the noni fruit
takes on an entirely
different appearance.

noninoninoninoninoninoninoninoninoninoni

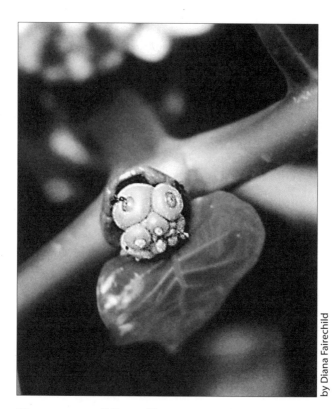

by Diana Fairechild

BIRTH OF A NONI FRUIT

Noni fruit pop out between a pair of leaves; this photo shows only one leaf next to the emerging noni, but there are always two leaves.

Fruit trees flower before they bear fruit. But not the noni tree—at least in appearance.

On noni trees, the fruit comes first, birthing between a pair of leaves. And then the flowers blossom on top of the fruit!

The fruit that pops out between a pair of noni leaves is actually called a receptacle, a fleshy base on which the flowers grow—so, technically, the fruit does not come before the flower.

Since many flowers grow on each noni receptacle, their developing ovaries clump together forming a composite fruit. Raspberries, figs and breadfruit are other examples of composite fruits. Oranges and apples are not composite fruits—they have single ovaries.

Noni flowers are described as "perfect," containing both male (pollen bearing) and female (ovary bearing) parts. Noni flowers are also very unusual in that some of the flowers have five petals and others have six petals, even on the same receptacle. [See the flowers on page 146.]

After each noni flower withers and drops off, a mark is left in its place on the receptacle.

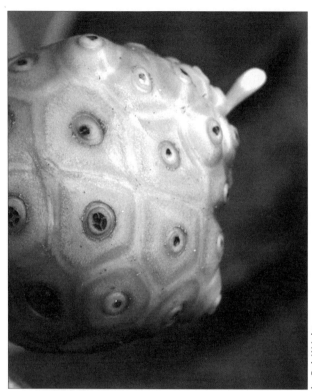

by Bob Wright

NONI GEOMETRY

Each "eye" is framed in a geometric ridge; a pentagon or hexagon reflecting the five-petal and six-petal flowers.

NONI by Diana Fairechild

It is obvious why these marks are known as noni "eyes." Around every eye a geometric frame develops—both pentagons and hexagons reflecting the five-petal and six-petal flowers. The photo, opposite, shows a green, or unripe, noni fruit with the geometric frames around the eyes. Also note the single flower bud at the top right.

The repetitive geometric frames and eyes remind me of the Louis Vuitton luggage logo; although the Vuitton luggage logo is perfectly repetitive, while the noni patterns are definitely not perfect. Sometimes the frames overlap, the pointy corners round into curves and soften into blurs. Noni patterns remind me of my own blurs (perceived imperfections) making the fruit seem friendly to me.

Noni flowers bloom on the side of the receptacle that gets the most sun. As the noni fruit matures it becomes lighter in color—from dark green to a bright greenish-yellow, then whitish-yellow, and finally the ripe fruit turns white with a human flesh-like transparency.

Mature noni has been described in medical and scientific research papers as a hand grenade, a wart, and a strange ovoid fruit.[5, 6, 7] These labels remind me how we tend to describe the

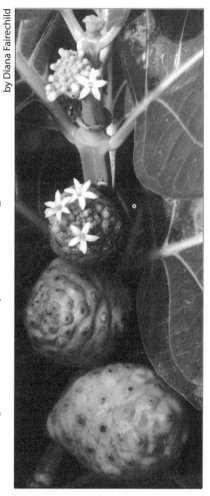

by Diana Fairechild

FIVE NONI BRANCH
Noni fruit grows horizontally in rows along the branches.

Noni bud

Noni receptacle with flowers

Two flowers have six petals and one has five

Green noni

Yellow noni

NONI by Diana Fairechild

world in terms that reflect our own inward conditions. The researcher who saw a hand grenade may have served in the military. The person who envisioned a wart may have been a doctor. A former flight attendant like myself *would certainly* see luggage logos!

On noni trees, the fruit—in all stages of maturity—grows in rows on the branches. Buds, flowers, unripe noni and ripe noni all grow one next to the other. [See opposite and page 148.]

. . . . It is early morning and I head down to the valley—looking for noni. *Thank you* I silently acknowledge each noni tree as I snap off the fruit. *Ba-bump* the fruit drums as I drop each piece into the bucket. *Ba-bump. Ba-bump. Thank you for being so fruitful even though no one is watering you. Thank you for healing me. The* morning light is increasing and the birds sing their exuberant welcome to this day. *Tweet-tweet woop-woop* I sing back mimicking their tunes.

As I pick the noni fruit, the little bud faces smile and promise me that when I come back next week and next month there will again be plenty of fruit to harvest—plenty of noni for detoxification and healing.

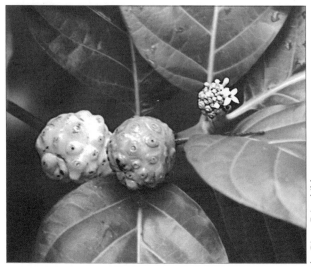

by Diana Fairechild

THREE NONI ON A BRANCH

From left: almost-ripe noni, green noni, flowering receptacle. Noni fruit grows in rows, outward from the trunk of the tree towards the ends of the branches.

Chapter 21
From Seed to Tree

noninoninoninoninoninoninoninoninoninoni

The properties
of a noni seed
and several suggested
planting methods.

noninoninoninoninoninoninoninoninoninoni

Behind the noni eyes there are seeds encased in a white jelly-like sac—similar to the pericardium that surrounds the precious hearts of humans.

Noni seeds are approximately the size of apple seeds and they are buoyant and can float hundreds of miles in the ocean and still be viable.

Noni seeds are easy to sprout. After preparing sun tea from the noni fruit, I take the leftover pulp and seeds and simply place it all in a plastic garden pot. At the bottom of the pot, I put some dirt mixed with potting soil, then the noni seeds, and over that more dirt so that the noni smell does not attract flies. Watered every day, the pot eventually fills up with bright green sprouts, which I sometimes harvest for salads.

It actually takes two months for noni seeds to germinate according to Karin Rosenberger, plant propagator at the Pacific Tropical Botanical Gardens on Kauai.

Noni trees can grow in either shade or sun—but sun-grown noni is 100-200% larger.

A farmer I know on Maui has thousands of wild noni trees on his property. Most of them are under the forest canopy. A couple of years ago, George moved several hundred 3-foot to 4-foot trees to higher ground where there is more sun because he found that fruit ripened in the sun is significantly larger; some of his noni fruits weigh up to a pound and a half.

One day I was visiting when George was digging up his small noni trees with his backhoe. Each noni tree has basically just a single root, called a taproot; there is no massive root system as with most trees. The taproots on the small noni trees were an inch and a half in diameter and about the same length as the tree height.

The ends of some of the roots broke off while George was digging them up, and I could see the interior of the roots—a yellow color that surprised me because it was so very bright.

It faded fast, though. The broken pieces of roots I took home with me faded in two days from the bright yellow to a dull pale ochre.

I have since learned that traditional Polynesian artists use the bright yellow color from the heart of the noni root, along with a red color from the noni bark, for dyeing tapa cloth.

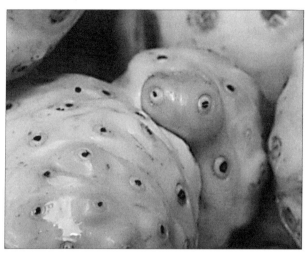

by Bob Wright

NONI SHMOO

Nestled among this noni crop was one small fruit, which appeared to look up at me and say, *Am I a noni or a shmoo? It's entirely up to you.*

Since noni fruit became a commercial crop George began to harvest his wild trees. From fifty trees he harvests approximately 550 pounds of fruit and gets 50 cents a pound; he picks his trees twice a month.

George said he saw no pests either in the noni fruit or in the roots. But a year later, the fruit on the small dug-up trees which had been replanted in rows as a commercial mono crop, was infested with a fungus Hawaiian farmers are calling "sooty mold"; and George had to treat his new noni orchard with a chemical.

On the Big Island, Kimo lives on family land with seventy-year-old noni trees that are forty feet tall. The land is in Kalapana where only five houses survived the 1990 lava eruption that dev-astated over a hundred homes. Even in drought times Kimo's noni trees produce fruit because the noni roots tap into an underground water source that is close to the surface.

In the process of pruning the old noni trees, Kimo found that he could simply stick an 18-inch long branch into a pot of soil and start a new tree. After about a year, these new trees were bearing fruit.

However, because the root structure of noni trees started from branches is lateral, not the single taproot, noni trees started from branches require about three times more water.

"No research has been done yet to determine whether the fruit from the trees with taproots have any different medicinal property than the fruit from the trees with lateral roots," says Scott, a producer of noni juice who buys the fruit from growers on all the Hawaiian Islands.

Scott also said that the noni trees growing among other types of trees are generally happier than the noni grown as a mono crop.

The reason, Scott believes, is that the noni trees love the "nutritional input from other fruit trees such as avocado, lichee, mangosteen and coconut as their fruit falls near by."

Noni trees grow companionably with many other types of fruit trees because the noni has no problem with root competition. The noni roots go deeper than forever, says Scott, as they tap down as far as they need to go to get water.

Scott also says that when the noni fruit is picked every two weeks this stimulates the trees into producing more noni.

On Maui, about a half mile from downtown Wailuku in a residential area, there is a 15-foot noni tree growing right above a cesspool. The tree's taproot is apparently accessing the contents of the cesspool and the fruit on this tree is the largest seen anywhere in the Hawaiian Islands, weighing over two pounds apiece.

It is not a tree I personally would want to pick from because of its nutrient source, but this clearly show how noni's taproot—like a hollow straw—sucks up whatever nutrient source is available.

Of course, noni assimilates whatever is in the surrounding soil as well. In this regard, Hawaiians with high blood pressure won't eat the noni that grows near the ocean because of its saline water source. It is also well known that it is unwise to eat noni from trees that are chemically fertilized.

In Kamaili on the Big Island, Nora is growing an orchard of organic noni. Every tree has been started from seed because Nora finds that trees started from seed develop the strongest taproot. "During droughts," says Nora, "the noni may stop producing fruit, but when there is a strong taproot, the leaves stay green and the trees remain healthy."

Nora began planting her noni in rows as is done in traditional fruit orchards; but then, one day, she got the idea that the noni did not want to be planted in rows one by one but rather as triads—three trees close together.

"As the noni trees mature, the branches get especially heavy because the fruit is growing farther and farther away from the trunk," Nora explained. "So when several noni trees are planted close together, the branches actually help to support each other—the trees hold each other's arms up."

I have noticed that noni trees have a way of pruning themselves, too, such that when the branches get too weighty with fruit, they break. When the lower branches are naturally trimmed back this way, the trees provide excellent shade.

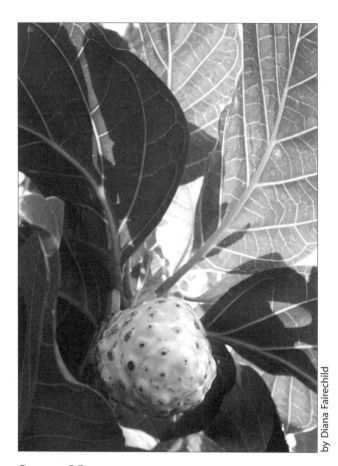

by Diana Fairechild

SHADY NONI

Noni leaves backlit by the sun.

NONI by Diana Fairechild

Chapter 23

Questions about Taking Noni

How do you
find noni products
and can you take
too much noni?

Questions About Taking Noni

How can you find noni products that are commercially made? Do you feel they are effective?

Noni is available in health food stores as juice, capsules, tea and tinctures. And many companies are selling noni on the Web.

In the preparation of noni, one's attitude while handling the noni plant is as important as the method of preparation. Keeping this in mind, I understand that some of the commercial noni products are made in a way that is careful, thoughtful, and reverent. And others may not be.

I have little experience with the commercial products and so I do not feel qualified to comment on them.

I believe, however, that we all have the power within ourselves to know if something is of value to us.

So I advise people to do research on the Internet or at a health food store and see which noni product you might feel like trying. Then, after you try a new product, give it a little time and regularly ask yourself: *Is this good for me?*

Can you overdose on noni and are there any bad side effects with noni?

This was something that concerned me as well when I first started using noni. I was attracted to noni because it has a long history of success without apparent toxic side effects.

Having been ill for a long time, I did not want to do anything that could possibly cause me harm.

"Side effects" is a very strong term. As I understand it, when pharmaceuticals are tested, the potential side effects are listed because too much of a pharmaceutical drug can be toxic.

Herbs are not tested in this way because they are not poisonous to begin with.

Yet I have found with noni that there are times when my symptoms seem to stir up so much that I have to back off from using it—sometimes for a few days, and sometimes even for a number of months.

I believe this is a very important part of healing with noni.

Is it okay for me to take noni while I'm taking other medicines?

Among Hawaiians, I'm told, it is known that people never take noni and pharmaceuticals at the same time because, taken together, neither will work.

In some way, noni neutralizes pharmaceuticals and noni appears to be rendered ineffective by pharmaceuticals.

Will unsterilized noni develop fungus or bacteria if stored for long periods of time?

No. According to testing, the older the noni the less fungal and bacteria growth it has.

Noni is not a favorable medium for fungus or bacteria because noni's pH is so low.

In fact, the fermentation process of noni neutralizes bacteria; one-year-old unpasteurized noni juice has a natural plant alcohol content of 1.45%, compared to beer which generally has 6% alcohol or wine which has 12% alcohol.

Does heating noni fruit destroy its medicinal properties?

Yes. Noni fruit heated over 110 degrees Fahrenheit, the maximum temperature noni will reach in its own natural environment, is known to be less effective medicinally because heat reduces noni's enzyme count.

Noni fruit can be commercially dried at 110 degrees, but higher temperatures translate into lowered enzymes.

A more starchy (rather than fruity and cheesy) taste identifies noni that has been dried at a high temperature.

Pasteurized noni juice is prepared at 160 to 190 degrees. Freeze-dried noni is prepared at up to 160 degrees.

Unpasteurized noni is not heated and it will continue to ferment even after it is bottled, becoming bubbly like champagne. To stop this fermentation process, add a small amount of apple cider vinegar to the noni juice.

In addition to its medicinal enzymes, noni contains many other active compounds (polysaccharides) believed to be responsible for noni fruit's medicinal efficacy.

It is not known how heat affects these other active compounds because not all of these compounds have yet been identified, much less tested.

Is noni safe to drink noni if it is prepared without sterilization?

The noni I drink, and have been drinking for five years with increasing positive results, is prepared without sterilization.

I put the washed, ripe fruit in closed jars in the sun for up to a year.

Once I open the jars and strain the seeds and skin, I keep the juice refrigerated and I believe my refrigerated noni is fine for up to another year.

One thing to consider, however, is to make sure your noni juice does not have any contact with metal because noni is known to oxidize metal. So don't use jars with metal lids either in the sun or in the refrigerator; metal lids will get rusty and then the flavor of the noni will become metallic.

Acknowledgments

noninoninoninoninoninoninoninoninoninoninoni

With heartfelt appreciation
I acknowledge these friends
who have helped me
to complete this book.

noninoninoninoninoninoninoninoninoninoninoni

Acknowledgments

Thanks to Kahalewai Ho'opai, who introduced me to noni. Bully, as he is known by his friends and eight thousand relatives around the Hawaiian Islands, healed himself from pesticide poisoning with noni juice. Kahalewai: "Everything is according to how you feel. If you feel good, keep taking it. If you feel nothing, but okay, keep taking it."

Thanks to Yvonne Conner, M.D. for encouraging me to try noni. Dr. Conner: "I don't see noni as having a bad taste. I see it as medicine. It's not ice cream, after all."

Thanks to Reverend Nani Saffery for information about diabetes. Nani: "It's the medicine and God together. I say this prayer every morning: God protect me through this day that I may stay well and strong."

Thanks to Dove White for sparking an interest in noni with her "Canoe Plants" column <hawaii-nation.org/canoe> and for her helpful and creative editorial assistance. Dove: "I hope the cultivators of noni work in a sacred manner, so that its healing properties are kept in tact."

Thanks to *kahuna* Lyons Kapi`ioho Naone for his interest in this project. Lyons: "There is no right way when it comes to using plants for traditional Hawaiian healing. Because it works, that's why we do it a certain way. On different islands we have different uses for the same plants and they may not agree with each other."

Thanks to Karin Rosenberger, plant propagator, and Rick Hanna, librarian, at the Pacific Tropical Botanical Garden. Thanks to Mary Lou Kelly at the Garden, who believed in this project at its earliest stage. Mary Lou: "Karin called and asked, 'How can Diana write a book if she doesn't know about propagating noni?' I answered, 'Diana's writing a different kind of book.'"

Special thanks to Patricia and Joseph Hanwright—who cherish the noni and propagate it—for being such good friends to noni and to me. Joseph "Joey Noni Seed" Hanwright: "I honor of the ancient Hawaiians and their gods."

Thanks to the following friends who helped with my research: Joe Licona (on car engines), Liz Lipsky (on ice cream), Frances Frazier (about ancient Hawaiians) and Joseph Kohlhepp (for rounding out the surfing metaphor). Joseph: "Allow yourself to be open, absorbing the power."

Thanks to Cynthia Wilson of the Chemical Injury Information Network for assistance in compiling the list of illnesses tracked to toxins. Cynthia: "Corporate multinationals have a vested interest in maintaining the fiction that chemical poisoning is psychological rather than a valid physiological response to their products."

Thanks to Joseph Ryan and Paul Wood for reading the manuscript and to Nina Anderson for reading the manuscript several times and for taking my photo with the noni. Nina: "Noni is the tree of life."

Thanks to Nora Freil and Kimo Blackenfeld for information about growing noni, Chuck and Nan Tipple for technical support, Bob Wright for capturing noni on film the way I was seeing it in the wild, Peter Waldo for looking at the noni under a microscope, and David Bylund for digitally preparing the illustrations for this edition. David: "These images make the noni seem so surreal; they have such a riveting presence."

Thanks to Rich Lafond and Roger Silber for insightful and essential editorial assistance and to Roger for assisting me with my mission in many wondrous ways. Rich: "Play with wonder, play with joy; inspire someone, especially yourself."

Deep appreciation to Scott Schuett for generously sharing information on growing noni and for escorting me around the Big Island. Scott: "I think noni is the most interesting plant. It grows in the hardest places—its roots penetrate lava—and it helps people with the hardest health problems."

Thanks to Anne MacAlpin for taking me to Kalapana and for taking the photo with the Kalapana noni. Please call; I've lost your number.

Thank you George Ewing, M.D., for coming to my aid when I was ill. You saved my life. How can I thank you? Dr. Ewing: "Keep climbing up the ladder. If you miss a rung, if you slip, just jump up and catch the next one."

Thanks to my dearest friends Peter and Dave Sanford who helped me to move to Hawaii. When I became ill, they never gave up on the idea that I would get my health back. Thank you for reading the manuscript many times. Thanks for your enthusiasm for this project! Peter: "I never had a swim I didn't like."

Endnotes

noninoninoninoninoninoninoninoninoninoni

Readers can use
these Endnotes for
further research and also
when referring to the
Table starting on
page 128.

noninoninoninoninoninoninoninoninoninoni

Endnotes

[1] *Our Toxic Times*, Jan. 1995, p. 16, Chemical Injury Information Network, P.O. Box 301, White Sulphur Springs, MT 59645.

[2] Monroe, Jason, Ph.D., "Urban Pesticide Control," *Our Toxic Times*, Sept. 1994, p. 1.

[3] Donnay, Albert, "Florida State Legislature," *Recognition of Multiple Chemical Sensitivity*, Nov. 1994, p. 5, MCS Referral and Resources, 506 Westgate Road, Baltimore, MD 21229.

[4] Kaiahua, Kalua with Noyes, Martha H., *Hawaiian Healing Herbs, a book of recipes*, 1997, Ka'imi Pono Press, Honolulu, HI.

[5] Tabrah, F.L., Hawaii Medical Journal, "Evaluation of Ancient Hawaiian Medicine," Vol. 25, 1966, pp. 223-230.

[6] Krauss, B., "Medicine and Medicinal Herbs," *Plants in Hawaiian Culture*, University of Hawaii Press, 1993, pp. 103, 252.

[7] Neal, M., *In Gardens of Hawaii*, Bishop Museum Press, Honolulu, HI, 1965, p 804.

[8] Stewart, Maria, "Noni, the Lore of Hawaiian Medicinal Plants," *The Bulletin*, Pacific Tropical

Botanical Garden, Kauai, HI, April 1972.

[9] Heinicke, R.M., *The Bulletin*, "The Pharmacologically Active Ingredient of Noni," Pacific Tropical Botanical Garden, Kauai, HI, Feb. 1985.

[10] Krauss, *Plants in Hawaiian Culture*, Ibid.

[11] Abbott, I.A., *La'au Hawaii: Traditional Hawaiian Uses of Plants, Medicines and Healing*, Bishop Museum Press, Honolulu, HI, 1992, pp. 97-100.

[10] Ibid.

[12] *Webster's New World Dictionary.*

[13] Elliott, Stephen and Brimacombe, Joseph "Medicinal Plants of Gunung Leuser National Park, Indonesia, *Journal of Ethnopharmacology*, Vol. 19, 1987, Elsevier Scientific Publishers Ireland, Ltd., pp. 285-317.

[14] Quisembing, E., "Medicinal Plants of the Philippines," Technical Bulletin, Vol. 16, 1951, Republic of the Philippines.

[15] Singh, Y. et al, "Folk Medicine in Tonga: A Study on the Use of Herbal Medicines for Obstetric and Gynecological Conditions and Disorders," Journal of Ethnopharmacology, Vol. 12, 1984, pp. 305-325.

[16] Whistler, W.A., "Tongan Herbal Medicine," *Isle Botanica*, Honolulu, HI, 1992, pp. 89-90.

[17] Tabrah, F.L., "Evaluation of the Effectiveness of Ancient Hawaiian Medicine," Ibid.

[18] Bushnell, O.A., Fukuda, M., Makinodan, T., "The Antibacterial Properties of Some Plants Found in Hawaii," Pacific Science, July 1950, pp. 167-183.

[19] Krauss, *Plants in Hawaiian Culture*, Ibid.

[20] Abbott, I.A. and Shimazu, C., "Geographic Origin of Plants Most Commonly Used for Medicine by Hawaiians," Journal of Ethnopharmacology, Vol. 14, 1985, pp. 213-222.

[21] Levand, O. and Larson, H.O., "Some Chemical Constituents of Morinda Citrifolia," Planta Med., Vol. 36, 1979, pp. 186-187.

[22] Whistler, W.A. "Traditional and Herbal Medicine in the Cook Islands," *Journal of Ethnopharmacology*, 1985, pp. 239-280.

[23] Heinicke, R.M., *The Bulletin*, Ibid.

[24] Hiramatsu, Tomonori, et al, "Induction of normal phenotypes in ras-transformed cells by Morinda Citrifolia," *Cancer Letters 73*, Keio Uni-

versity, Japan, 1993, pp. 161-166.

[25] Hirazumi, A., "Antitumor Activity of Morinda Citrifolia on Lung Carcinoma in Mice," American Association for Cancer Research, Vol. 33, Mar. 1992, p. 515.

[26] Douglass, Dr. William Campbell, "Second Opinion," Atlanta, GA, 10-97, p. 8.

[27] Steingraber, Sandra, PhD, "Living Down-stream: Cancer and the Environment," *Canary News*, Vol. 46, 1997, Evanston IL 60201.

[28] Carr, Clark, "The Impact of the Detoxification Program," *FASE Research*, Foundation for Advancements in Science, Los Angeles, CA 90010.

[29] Handy, E., Kawena Pukui, M. Livermore, K., "Outline of Hawaiian Physical Therapeutics," Bishop Museum, Bulletin 126, Honolulu, 1934.

[30] Kaaiakamanu, D.M., Akina, J.K., "Hawaiian Herbs of Medicinal Value," Pacific Books, 1922.

[31] McBride, L.R., *Practical Folk Medicine of Hawaii*, Petroglyph Press, 1975, p. 55.

Books, Consulting, Presentations

noninoninoninoninoninoninoninoninoninoni

Perhaps you would
like to contact Diana
or find out more about
her other activities.

noninoninoninoninoninoninoninoninoninoni

Books by Diana Fairechild

NONI: Aspirin of the Ancients

3rd Edition, Revised and Updated, 2001
The lore and the lure of this powerful, ancient plant.

NONI, autographed, $9.95
Shipping/Handling, $4.50 U.S./$9 international

OFFICE YOGA: At-Your-Desk Exercises

You can prevent painful back, neck and wrists, as well as headaches and fuzzy thinking caused by sitting for long hours at a computer. For your body to function optimally, you need to make regular adjustments in your behavior. Bodily adjustments can also be made by physicians, chiropracters and massage therapists. If you self-correct with the help of a healer or on your own, you can usually catch misalignments before they cause you downtime or long-term harm. Self-correction is a synonym for "yoga."

"Clearly written, thoroughly illustrated, this book is a treasure for anyone who works at a desk."—*Kauai Magazine*

"Fairechild's *Office Yoga* is a wonderful, thoughtful, practical guide for working professionals to help them improve their concentration and thus be more productive at work."—Arthur Brownstein, M.D., Holistic Medicine

OFFICE YOGA, autographed, $9.95
Shipping/Handling, $4.50 U.S./$9 international

JET SMARTER: The Air Traveler's Rx

There are dangers in air travel, some obvious, many hidden. The air in commercial jets is toxic. And the oxygen is inadequate—pilots get ten times more than passengers. Pesticides are sprayed on seats, on luggage, and sometimes right on passengers. Radiation for frequent flyers equals that of atomic energy workers. Drawing on 21 years' experience as an airline insider, Fairechild gives readers a rare, no-holds-barred look at the dangers of air travel and offers hundreds of sensible ways to cope with or even avoid their impact on one's health. JET SMARTER can startle readers with how hazardous airline practices are, comfort readers with the author's personally-tested approach to surviving the air travel experience, and entertain readers with Diana Fairechild's sometimes gentle, sometimes gritty, but always grand sense of humor.

"Thanks, Diana. You're doing great work. I refer many to your book. All are amazed and grateful for its contents."—David Stenn, screenwriter

"Fairechild discusses all the health hazards endemic to airline travel."—Andrew Weil, M.D.

"Take the advice of Diana Fairechild."—*Smart Money*

JET SMARTER, autographed, $14.95
Shipping/Handling $4.50 U.S./$10 international

Consulting & Photographs

FEARLESS FLYER CONSULTING

Are you afraid to fly? Fearless Flyer will transform your fear of flying—with warmth, with humor, and with simple, powerful strategies. A personal phone consultation with Diana Fairechild is a quick and economical way to clear your fear of flying."

> "Within five minutes on the phone with you, I knew things were going to change. The skills you gave me for flying are life skills that transcend to all other areas of my life. You have given me a gift, and I thank you so much."
> —*Beth Farmer, homemaker*

Email or Call for Phone Appointment
Hourly Consulting Rate

FULL COLOR 8" x 12" NONI PHOTOS

Imagine the photos in this book in full color. The micro-photography allows you to intimately know the noni tree.

"Bee Into Noni Flower" (page 64)
"Five Noni Branch" (page 144)
"Noni Bud Face" (page 72 and front cover)
"Noni Flower" (page 60)
"Noni Leaf" (page 108)

Full Color 8" x 12" Noni Photos, $20 each
Shipping/Handling, $4.50 U.S./ $10 int'l per order

The Fair Air Coalition

The Fair Air Coalition is a tax-exempt, non-profit advocacy organization run by airline passengers for the benefit of airline passengers. Many of the challenging conditions of air travel that compound jetlag and risk passengers' health and peace of mind are preventable. What is required is that the airlines come to understand that passengers are willing to stand up for health as an issue of airline safety.

Personally, I have been an advocate for airline passengers since the publication of my first book, JET SMART, in 1992. The book took me fourteen years to write, so, at this point it's fair to say that my commitment to improving conditions for airline passengers officially began in 1978.

In 1997, I founded The Fair Air Coalition as a Hawaii Domestic Nonprofit Corporation, ID 99-0332878 to help me continue this work.

The Fair Air Coalition is presently involved in focusing media attention on aviation health issues and educating legislators and the flying public on flight-induced maladies. Any donation or involvement is gratefully accepted. Thank you.

Diana Fairechild, director
The Fair Air Coalition
PO Box 248, Anahola Hawaii 96703—USA

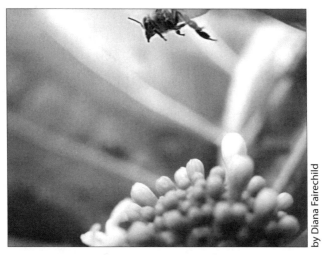

by Diana Fairechild

BEE COMMUNING WITH NONI

How wonderous the noni must look and smell to the bees.

Speaking

Diana Fairechild teaches seminars to groups and corporations on minimizing the ill effects of jet travel and maximizing productivity and efficiency after flying. She also speaks on the subjects of detoxification, office yoga, self publishing., and fear of flying. Fairechild has been quoted by *Forbes, Smart Money, USA Today, The National Law Journal, Whole Earth Review* and CNN. She is the author of four books and has also written freelance for ABCNews.com and Reuters News Service. Prior to writing and speaking, she served as an international flight attendant for 21 years, flying 10 million miles around the world. Arrange for Diana Fairechild to speak to your group anywhere in the world. Her enthusiasm is inspiring. For easy to follow, engaging presentations, call 808/828-1919.

"Members will not want to board another plane until they've heard what Diana Fairechild has to say."
—*American Board of Trial Advocates*

"It is magical to see so many writers, all with different projects at different levels of doneness, and watch their books come to fruition in Diana's course. The classes are interactive, so they take on a life of their own."
—*J. Van Pelt, Executive, Kauai Electric*

Comments from
Readers & Editors

noninoninoninoninoninoninoninoninoninoni

Feel free to send
your comments
for possible inclusion
in future editions.

noninoninoninoninoninoninoninoninoninoni

"This paean to noni and its curative powers is written in the same humorous, quirky, whimsical style as Diana Fairechild's first book, JET SMART. It provides fascinating reading about this little-known fruit, including photos, recipes, and instructions for its use. Best of all, perhaps, it gives one the feeling of a short trip to the good air and relaxed living of those wonderful islands in the Pacific. Try it."

—*Lynn Lawson*
CanaryNews, Evanston, Illinois

"If you read this book you'll want to grow a noni tree in your back garden! Diana has gathered a great deal of information on this fruit and, in an easily read style, has explained and shown how to use the Morinda Citrifolia tree to benefit you and your loved ones' health. Diana's bibliography shows how many others know of the healing benefits of noni, and almost every chapter describes a new way of using the tree, and especially the juice. I read the book twice within the first few days. I highly recommend it."

—*Alan G. Clark*
London, England

"I just finished NONI. Loved it! Picked it up at Borders last night and finished it up zip-zip today. I was moved to tears. The surfing metaphor is right on. I am enrolled in having a personal relationship with noni, too. Thanks for your great contribution with this book. I plan to share it with many."

—Dee Dowdy
San Francisco, California

"I read your NONI book and I could not put it down until I was done. It was exhilarating, spiritual and very moving at the same time. Thanks."

—Judy Haroldson
Orange County, California

"Diana Fairechild has put together the most complete writing on noni—culturally and spiritually— that I have ever seen."

—Lyons Kapiioho Naone
Maui Kahuna, Hawaii

"I am impressed with Diana Fairechild's NONI. I like the humor and satire. I would like to prescribe noni to my patients."

—Vincent Mark, M.D.
Environmental Medicine, Santa Cruz, California

"After I was diagnosed with severe, chronic asthma and told I would have to take steroids for the rest of my life, I began to listen more to my body, and I came across your book. Since then, I can successfully declare myself healed of asthma. If I do feel congested, the noni immediately clears it up. I always use your recipe for preparing fresh noni. Thank you for your insightful book on healing with noni. What a sacred, odd, lovable, wonderful little fruit. *Mahalo nui loa* for sharing your *mana`o* with me."

—*Angelique Tepper, Haleiwa, Hawaii*

"On a visit to the health food store, your NONI book jumped up into my arms—and I am forever thankful. A quarter-sized boil had grown along my spine. All I had to go on were the pictures in your book. One morning, as I was jogging, something made my feet slow down and marched me straight over to a noni tree! I was stunned! Suddenly I recognized many noni trees all around me and I became quite excited. I felt as if a prayer had been answered. I decided to try the noni leaves on the boil. After one day there was no pain. After a few days the boil was gone."

—*Kari Meadow, Big Island*

"Thank you for sending out your book so fast. It arrived in the afternoon mail and I am only now finishing it. It's 1:00 am and I feel like I just surfed a perfect wave. When I first drank noni juice, the release of toxins made me feel a little sick. Now, after reading your book, I will quit using it for a week and allow my body to rest."

—*Kirk Hamilton*

"Received your wonderful book today. Thank you so much for the personal autograph. I have been taking noni since 1996 and agree completely with you that it is wonderful. I was diagnosed with breast cancer on December 23rd, 1994."

—*Diana Morrell*

"I just finished reading NONI and loved it, especially your sense of humor. Hope you are doing well. I have just barely begun to practice what you explain as the most important part of healing: the gut feelings, the waking up, following your heart, and being responsible for yourself. It is a good beginning. I wish you well and pray for healing for all who are seeking it."

—*Etti, Kihei, Hawaii*

For More Information
Contact Diana Fairechild

Email	diana@flyana.com
Web	www.flyana.com
Phone	808/828-1919
Write	PO Box 248
	Anahola Hawaii
	96703–USA

Books

Consulting

Presentations